Computer Applications in Mental Health: Education and Evaluation

Computer Applications in Mental Health: Education and Evaluation

Marvin J. Miller
Editor

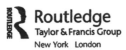

Routledge
Taylor & Francis Group
New York   London

Routledge is an imprint of the
Taylor & Francis Group, an informa business

Computer Applications in Mental Health: Education and Evaluation, has also been published as *Computers in Human Services*, Volume 8, Numbers 3/4 1992.

Reprinted 2009 by Routledge

Library of Congress Cataloging-in-Publication Data

Computer applications in mental health : education and evaluation / Marvin J. Miller, editor.
    p.   cm.
    "Has also been published as Computers in human services, volume 8, numbers 3/4 1992" – T.p. verso.
    Includes bibliographical references.
    ISBN 1-56024-279-5 (alk. paper). – ISBN 1-56024-353-8 (pbk. : alk. paper)
    1. Mental health – Data processing – Congresses. 2. Psychiatry – Data processing – Congresses. I. Miller, Marvin J., 1946- .
    [DNLM: 1. Computers – congresses. 2. Information Systems – congresses. 3. Mental Health – congresses. 4. Psychiatry – methods – congresses. W1 CO457YC v. 8 no. 3/4 / WM 26.5 C7378]
RA790.5.C645 1992
362.2'0285'53 – dc20
DNLM/DLC
for Library of Congress
                                        92-1541
                                           CIP

Computer Applications in Mental Health: Education and Evaluation

Computer Applications in Mental Health: Education and Evaluation

CONTENTS

Computer Applications in Mental Health: Education and Evaluation

ABOUT THE EDITOR

Marvin J. Miller, MD, is an Assistant Professor of Psychiatry at Indiana University School of Medicine. He is a research psychiatrist at Larue Carter Hospital investigating issues of psychopharmacology and computer uses in psychiatry. He has also been chair of the Clinical Computing Committee for the Indiana Department of Mental Health and is a Member of the Information Systems Committee of the American Psychiatric Association. He was the organizer of the second annual meeting entitled "Computer Applications in Mental Health — 1991" held April 19, 1991 in Indianapolis, Indiana. All of the chapters in this book are revisions of material presented at that conference.

Preface

A conference entitled "Computer Applications in Mental Health – 1991 Update" was held in Indianapolis, Indiana on 04-19-91. The chapters in this book are all revisions of papers presented at that conference. The range of topics discussed included the large mental health package used within the Veteran's Administration Hospital system (costing millions) at one end of the spectrum and a variety of micro-computer applications (often funded by individuals) at the other end of the spectrum.

The field of mental health computing has moved past some early phases characterized by much optimism and large sums of Federal or State funding on to the current phases where different approaches predominate. Many current applications are implemented on low-cost micro-computers with software development funded at a very low level or through individual sweat and determination. The early optimism has been replaced by a more concrete, pragmatic need to focus on a very small area of computer application with the need to show validity and effectiveness in a defined topic.

A very welcome and promising spin-off of this new "small is beautiful" approach is the ability to share the software developed at little or no cost. Several of the packages discussed are available on computerized Bulletin Board Systems (BBS's) at no cost beyond that of a long distance phone call (see Chapter 2). Much information in the scientific community is freely shared with other professionals and other investigators. This philosophy is shared by many authors in this book.

The specific topics discussed include a very technical computerized analysis of speech patterns, a screening battery for community mental health centers, evaluation of suitable reinforcers for patients, as well as devices to speed up the processing of paper work within a large state hospital. Several aspects of patient education are also discussed. These topics will be of interest to a broad segment of mental health professionals and will hopefully stimulate further development and sharing of computer software.

Marvin J. Miller, MD

Mental Health
Clinical Computer Applications
That Succeed:
The VA Experience

Robert M. Kolodner

KEYWORDS. Software acceptance, mental health software, clinical applications

SUMMARY. Clinicians and researchers alike have been foretelling the arrival of the use of computers in mental health since the mid 1960's. Many of the applications that have been developed since that time were implemented at single sites or were developed in a research environment. Relatively few applications were implemented and used in the day-to-day care of patients at multiple facilities. The mental health software currently being used by the largest

---

Robert M. Kolodner, MD, is Assistant Director of Psychiatry at the Department of Veterans Affairs Medical Center at Dallas, TX and a member of the Department of Psychiatry at The University of Texas Southwestern Medical Center in Dallas, TX. Requests for reprints should be sent to Robert M. Kolodner, MD, Psychiatry Service (116A), VA Medical Center, 4500 South Lancaster Rd., Dallas, TX, 75216.

The author gratefully acknowledges the able and reliable assistance of Sylvia Hougland, MPA, who edited the paper and provided valuable input and of Lynn Carroll, who prepared this manuscript.

This paper was only possible due to the dedicated and diligent work by the members of the VA Mental Health Special Interest Users Group (SIUG) over the past eight years. Special thanks goes to those who survived the task of programming the software only to be subjected to the torrent of "small changes" requested by the eager group of users. These include Dr. Douglas Gottfredson and Deborah Price who were the Project Developers as well as the cadre of clinician-programmers who served on the SIUG: Drs. Alan Finkelstein, Marina Bates, Robert Lushene, and D. Robert Fowler.

1

number of clinicians at multiple facilities is the software developed in the Department of Veterans Affairs. This paper will review the lessons learned from the development and use of the software in VA settings. Both barriers and facilitating factors for implementation and adoption of mental health software will be identified as part of this review.

INTRODUCTION

Clinicians and researchers alike have been foretelling the arrival of the use of computers in mental health since the mid 1960's (American Psychiatric Association, 1969). Unfortunately, although we first thought that the applications would be "just around the corner," it has been a far more enterprising and tedious process to develop clinical applications than was first thought. There have been several excellent reviews of applications in mental health including some analyses of the problems associated with implementing these systems (Greist & Klein, 1981; Hedlund et al., 1981; Lieff, 1987; Schwartz, 1984; Sidowski, Johnson, & Williams, 1980).

Many of the applications reported in these reviews were implemented at single sites or were developed in a research environment. Relatively few computer applications were used in the day-to-day care of patients at multiple facilities (Glueck, 1974; Hedlund et al., 1981; Laska, 1976). All of the early, facility-based mental health computer systems have ceased to be used. Many of the systems involved either batch mode or clerical entry of data that provided feedback to the clinicians through paper documents generated by the system. Although they were state of the art at the time, they did not evolve into on-going systems.

The mental health software currently being used by the largest number of clinicians at multiple facilities is the software developed in the Department of Veterans Affairs (VA). This paper will discuss lessons learned from the development and use of this public domain software in VA settings. The experience in the VA complements and extends observations made earlier on the use of software by clinicians both in mental health and other disciplines (Hedlund et al., 1981). Both barriers to and facilitating factors for implementation and adoption of mental health software will be identified as part of this review.

HISTORY OF THE VA SOFTWARE

The VA Administration began implementing a large hospital information system in 1978. The system is now used in 167 VA medical facilities nationwide. The software has also been adapted for use in the Indian Health Service and in the Department of Defense Medical Facilities. The VA system, referred to as the Decentralized Hospital Computer Program (DHCP), is written in MUMPS language, can be run on almost any hardware platform, and is flexible enough to be used in a wide variety of clinical settings. The VA-wide dissemination of this system was facilitated by a Congressional mandate in 1982. The initial applications of Medical Administration, Laboratory and Pharmacy were installed in all facilities in 1985. Periodic upgrades in hardware at each facility have allowed an increasing number of applications to be supported at each site. The list of software packages currently available in DHCP is extensive (Table 1).

The VA's Mental Health System (MHS) was adapted from software first developed at Salt Lake City VA in the early 1970's (Johnson & Williams, 1975). The original software was subsequently modified and expanded at the Bay Pines and Dallas VA Medical Centers. In 1983, a group comprised of mental health clinicians, administrators, and computer specialists reviewed the existing software and identified changes necessary to generalize it for use throughout the VA. The software became available for nationwide use in 1985. However, until recently, most VA facilities either did not install the mental health software at all or did so on a restricted basis due to limitations in hardware availability.

The MHS continued to be improved under the direction of the VA's Mental Health Special Interest Users Group, and a subsequent version (4.0) was released in 1990. This second release included a number of enhancements. The diagnostic scheme was updated from DSM-III to DSM-III-R, progress notes were improved by adding the ability to electronically sign the notes and print them for inclusion in the medical record, and a set of Inpatient Features applica-

Table 1

VA DHCP Software
Clinical Management

Clinical Record
    Health Summary
    Order Entry /
        Results Reporting
Dentistry
Dietetics
Immunology Case Registry
Laboratory
    Anatomic Pathology
    Blood Bank
Medicine.
Mental Health
Nursing

Pharmacy
    Automatic Replenishment
    Inpatient Medications
    National Drug File
    Outpatient Pharmacy
Quality Assurance
    External Review
    Incident Reporting
    Occurrence Screen
    Utilization Review
Radiology
Social Work
Surgery

Administrative Management

Decentralized Medical/
    Management System
Diagnostic Related Grouper
Engineering
Fee Basis
Integrated Funds Control/
    Accounting and
        Procurement
    Accounts Receivable
    General Inventory
    Personal Funds of
    Patients
Interim Management Support
Library

Medical Administration
    Admission/Transfer/
      Discharge
    Automated Medical
    Discretionary Workload
    Hospital Inquiry
    Scheduling
Medical Care Cost/
    Recovery
Personnel and Accounting
    Integrated Data
    Personnel & Fiscal/
      Transactions
    Time and Attendance
Record Tracking

System/Database Management

Kernel
    Mailman
    VA Fileman

Letterman
VA Classman
VA Generic Code Sheet

For further information about software, contact the Hines
Information Systems Center, Department of Veteran's Affairs,
Bldg. 37, Hines, IL 60141. (708) 216-2197.

tions was added. The latter provides the ability to assign patients to
clinical teams and then to enter and retrieve information regarding
all of the patients on that team. This facilitates the delivery of care
to inpatients at sites where inpatient clinicians are organized into
interdisciplinary mental health teams.

The MHS is in the forefront of software designed for use by front-line clinicians in the VA. It preceded applications designed for Internal Medicine and Surgery, which have only recently been developed and released. With the arrival of new hardware, all VA facilities having a mental health program have implemented the MHS. The software is used by a wide variety of VA staff, including psychiatrists, psychologists, nurses, nursing assistants, social workers, physician assistants, residents, students, psych techs, administrators, clerks, and occupational and physical therapists. In addition to having access to the mental health software, these users have had the ability to retrieve laboratory, pharmacy, and radiology data through DHCP on patients they have been treating. Security is controlled in a better manner than the paper record, and the ability to access information is provided on a "need to know" basis. Experience at different hospitals has shown that there is a wide variation from site to site in the degree to which this system is used by clinicians and in the selection of applications that those clinicians use. The remainder of this paper focuses on the reasons for this variation.

DEFINING A SUCCESSFUL APPLICATION

The VA system differs from that of the private sector in that there is little financial pressure on individuals to use this system in order to get reimbursed. Use is generally driven by the utility of the software for the clinician and the commitment of the clinical administrators to encourage use of the system. There is little authority to coerce clinicians to use the software. VA clinicians have a great deal of individual discretion regarding whether or not they will use DHCP.

In order to identify computer applications that have been successfully implemented in the VA, one must define what constitutes being "successful." A successful application is one that is used voluntarily by many clinicians at numerous different sites. It is especially important that the applications be accepted and used routinely by clinicians at medical facilities beyond the initial development or test sites, since the presence of "champions" at these sites may disproportionately influence the use of the software.

This approach to defining success relies on clinicians to determine, by their behavior, what computer applications are most useful to them and seeks to identify those applications that can succeed in the absence of administrative efforts to mandate their use. It is also an important criterion that the software be used until it is replaced by another application that is better at meeting the needs of the user. An absence of "staying power" for an application may indicate that the hoped for achievements were not delivered over a period of time. Applications could also fade from use for other reasons, such as a change in user needs, or a degradation in computer system performance or support.

Additional factors at a site will be identified that may preclude the use of the software at all, thus preventing some clinicians from getting a chance to adequately test and either adopt or reject an application.

Primary emphasis will be placed on mental health computer applications. However, treating patients with psychiatric problems also involves the provision of general medical care. Thus, some of the successful applications listed are classified as part of a broader category than just mental health.

SUCCESSFUL APPLICATIONS

Clinicians appear to more readily accept applications with little or no required data entry. This is especially true for physicians, who are the clinicians most resistant to using and incorporating computers into their daily practice. Even so, many physicians routinely turn to a clerk to retrieve patient information rather than signing onto the computer and retrieving information. This trend may be changing as younger, computer literate physicians enter the field of medicine.

Data Retrieval

Some of the first applications installed in the VA hospitals involved laboratory and pharmacy services. Although the software was designed for managing the daily operation of those services, the by-product of this software was on-line retrieval of laboratory results and pharmacy prescriptions. Clinicians, including those in mental health, first used DHCP to look up patient demographic information as well as laboratory, pharmacy, and radiology results. This often required making two or three selections on different menus and re-entering the patient identification in order to retrieve such results.

Within the MHS, several retrieval applications have been widely used. The oldest and most successful of the applications is that of self-administered psychological tests and interviews. This application allows patients to directly interact with the computer and to respond to questions displayed on the screen by entering their responses with one or two keystrokes on a standard keyboard. The MHS contains 44 tests and 33 interviews that can be administered to patients by way of a standard computer terminal. Patients have been remarkably receptive to entering their responses directly into the computer. Clinicians then have both the raw information and the computer scoring available to them on-line. This sometimes includes an interpreted report, such as with the MMPI. Clinicians are receptive because of the accuracy and ease of scoring, the time savings in test administration, the flexibility to have clerk entry of test data, and the ability to append clinician comments to test results. Contracts have been written with the companies holding the copyright for those tests and interviews in the MHS not in the public domain.

An MHS application called "Profile of Patient" displays information regarding patient demographics, when the patient applied for care at the facility, admission and discharge dates for their last five hospitalizations, and a brief listing of the progress notes, physical exams, and histories that have been entered into the computer for the patient. A summary of the last physical examination is also available in this profile. This application has been well received at many of the sites. In the future, this application may be supplemented or replaced by the Health Summary application to be described below.

The "Inpatient Features" application provides capabilities to the inpatient mental health wards, which are subsets of the inpatient wards at most VA Medical Centers. A report can be obtained that indicates the number of operating beds, the current census, the number of empty beds, and the scheduled admissions for each mental health ward. The software provides each site with the ability to tailor this report for their individual needs. For example, wards can be clustered on the report so that the acute wards and rehabilitation wards can be sub-totalled separately. This application also provides the ability to define mental health teams, often organized around house staff or an attending physician. Patients can be assigned to the team responsible for their care. The team can then draw up a list of their patients whether on a single ward or across wards, and a work list can be printed with a variable amount of space between the patients names. Included on this work list are the each patient's name and identifier, age, date of hospital entry, current length of stay, and the primary diagnosis for which they are being treated. These sheets can be used to take notes during rounds or to sign out to other physicians for night call. Many nurses use these work lists at the time of nursing report to take notes regarding the patients on the ward. A variety of reports can be obtained about the team and about the patients treated by that team including lists of patients admitted or discharged during selected intervals, their diagnostic mix and length of stay. This ability to retrieve information about patients based on the team to which they are assigned, complements the standard Medical Administrative software used by the admission and ward clerks.

A recently developed application called Health Summary is just now being disseminated throughout the VA. Although Health Summary has not yet achieved those characteristics that define it as a successful application, it has been widely acclaimed in its early use at test sites. Preliminary indications are that it will be well received. Health Summary integrates test results as well as additional information such as discharge diagnoses, past and future appointments, and mental health progress notes into a single report. The application also allows the user to page forward and backward on a terminal while in the report and optionally print the report. A Customized Health Summary can be created to meet the specific needs of each hospital location (ICU, Surgical Ward, Emergency Room, Mental Health Clinic, Cardiology Clinic, etc.) or individual clinicians, so that the patient report that is displayed or printed fits the desired purpose. This builds on and extends the Profile of Patient option noted above and on other similar kinds of reports that have been created at non-VA sites (McDonald et al., 1984).

Data Entry

As mentioned previously, clinicians are often much more resistant to using computers for data entry tasks than for data retrieval alone. The most widely used application on DHCP for data entry is the electronic mail system. Although some users do not take advantage of this application, many others communicate extensively with their colleagues by using the VA electronic mail. The capability exists to send messages to any VA employee who has access to the computer at one of the 167 Medical Centers as well as to those at the Information Systems Centers, and the Regional and Central Offices. This networking across facilities provides a very powerful means for colleagues to communicate. The primary use for electronic mail remains that of communicating within a facility. The user composes his message using a very simple line editor provided by the VA software. There have been a number of complaints regarding the limitations of this primitive line editor, but despite these reservations, the electronic mail continues to be heavily utilized.

Serendipitously, electronic mail provides a very low pressure environment in which the clinicians can learn to use most of the features necessary for data entry in DHCP. Once users are facile with composing and sending electronic mail, they will have learned most of the conventions by all DHCP software. Thus, the electronic mail provides an ideal environment for the clinical users to practice the skills needed for use in general clinical data entry.

Within the MHS, the most widely used applications for data entry are the psychological test and interviews, usually entered by the patient but with some of the tests, such as the BPRS also entered by clinicians. Physical examination, DSM-III-R diagnoses and progress notes applications also require data entry by clinicians and are used extensively by clinicians at multiple VA facilities.

The physical examination application was one of the early programs developed at the Salt Lake VA Medical Center. It provides a very simple way to record a physical examination, often much more quickly than by handwriting the exam. The results are printed in a format that can be placed in the medical record after the clinician signs the printout. The report summarizes abnormal or omitted examinations at the top. A brief paragraph is then printed for each body system indicating the components of a normal exam, if the exam was normal. If the exam was not normal, it lists those portions that would be checked as part of a routine physical examination when abnormalities are noted.

At some facilities, the physical exam application is used extensively due to the ability to retrieve the results of the physical exam at any time, even when the chart is not available. The application is used even by medical students, who rotate through the facility for a very short 30-day rotation, because of the ease of data entry and rapidity of producing the report provided by the software. However, at other sites, no physical examinations are entered in the computer. This may be due to the limited number of terminals available, the lack of familiarity with the software capabilities, or clinicians' objections to the fixed narrative output.

Less extensively used are applications to enter DSM-III-R diagnoses and to record and print crisis and progress notes. The diagnosis routine allows for rapid entry of patients' clinical diagnoses that on all five axes of DSM-III-R. The first two axes are combined for data entry purposes and an extensively cross-referenced list of terms can be used to look up the appropriate diagnosis. The application requires a minimum of key strokes and no memorization on the part of the clinician regarding DSM-III-R numbers or which modifiers are required for any given diagnosis. For example, typing in "BIP MAN" will display a list of all DSM-III-R diagnoses regarding Mania. The software then leads the users through the entry of all necessary data. On-line help is available, including the definition of the scoring ranges for Axis V. This routine appears to be used more on inpatient than in outpatient settings because of the ability to review diagnosis for all patients on a clinical team. A similar retrieval of data can only be accomplished in the outpatient setting on a patient-by-patient basis. No report is printed by this application for inclusion in the chart.

Progress notes can be entered into the computer, signed electronically, and printed for inclusion in the medical record. Entry is accomplished through the use of the same standard DHCP editor used in electronic mail. This line editor does not provide for any spell checker or other more sophisticated supports for the user. In general, clinicians are reluctant to type free text into the computer. However, at a few sites clinicians have used progress notes extensively, especially in their outpatient settings, entering notes for up to 80% of outpatient visits. Once the notes are entered, they are available from any terminal in the facility even when the other medical record is not otherwise available. This facilitates continuity of care especially in outpatient settings for emergency situations or unscheduled visits.

A variation on the progress notes is the crisis note. This is a note which appears the first time a patient is selected each day by a user. This crisis note is used to alert the users about an important clinical situation regarding the patient. These include any suicidal or homicidal potential that the patient might have or other important factors to consider whenever the patient is treated or seen in an emergency setting. The current design of the VA system allows only the mental health users to see these messages. Users in other disciplines or outside of mental health do not have access. This feature will be expanded during the next year as the progress notes option is generalized for use by clinicians from all disciplines.

UNSUCCESSFUL APPLICATIONS

Most authors report on their successful or apparently successful applications. It is much more difficult to find examples of papers reporting unsuccessful efforts to implement. Within the MHS there are a couple of applications that have been used very infrequently during the time they have been available in the VA. It is particularly instructive to examine these unsuccessful applications in order to identify factors which may inhibit the distribution and use of available clinical software.

The first of these applications is the problem list. The design of this particular software is awkward for the clinicians to use in order to enter a problem on the list. In addition, the problem list does not print a version which can be placed in the chart and, thus, does not replace additional documentation that needs to be done in the paper record. The user must do separate entries in the computer and in the paper chart and work to keep both of these synchronized and up to date. Clinicians have chosen not to do the extra work and this problem list goes unused at the vast majority of sites.

A second partial application that is also not used because of clinical difficulties is that of Axis 3 diagnosis. Axis 3 involves the diagnoses of medical problems that coexist and influence diagnoses on Axes 1 and 2. The MHS software uses the existing ICD-9CM file used by the medical record coders who are administrative personnel. This software does not have extensive cross-referencing and is not organized in the way that clinical users think. For example, the software does not recognize commonly used clinical abbreviations such as "CVA" or "TIA" and will simply beep at the user if such abbreviations or clinical terms are used. An enhancement to this file was developed in the Indian Health Service to add an extensive list of terms used by clinicians in day-to-day practice and correlate these terms to specific ICD-9 diagnoses. This addendum might improve the clinical utility of acceptance of ICD-9 codes. However, this extension has not been available within the VA until recently, so no experience has been gained in the VA from such a change.

DISCUSSION

The six years of experience in the VA with the MHS, including the past year with the recently updated version, demonstrates and reinforces a number of principles and factors that appear to influence the acceptance of clinical software within Mental Health. Some of these factors have been cited by previous authors (Hedlund et al., 1981).

These factors appear to fall into two major categories: system factors and software factors. Each of these can be further subdivided into additional components.

SYSTEM FACTORS

System factors include both hardware and environmental elements. As demonstrated by the limited implementation of the MHS at most VA sites until recently, there must be adequate access to terminals and printers in order to utilize clinically-oriented software. Clinicians will not tolerate queuing up to use the terminal, especially if they are in a time limited patient interaction such as those encountered in outpatient clinics. The computer may be able to integrate existing data in a clinically usable, but non-interactive, form if summary reports can be generated prior to the clinical encounter. This is one way that the Health Summary may be used in clinical settings. The original mental health software was not designed to generate such outputs ahead of time except for the Inpatient Team lists which have received some broad acceptance on the inpatient wards when they have been available.

If the user is expected to interact in "real" time with the computer system, then the software response time must also be "tolerable." The limits for this tolerability vary depending on what the user is attempting to do. If they are doing data entry, then the response time must be almost instantaneous or the user will quickly get frustrated and stop attempting to perform data entry functions. Generating a summary report across patients can take longer without the user rejecting the system.

Environmental factors play a significant role in how many individuals at the site use the software. The phenomenon of a clinical gatekeeper or a local "champion" has been noted at a number of the sites. The presence of such local champions is helpful in facilitating the dissemination and adoption of the clinical software into daily care but it does not ensure success. Some sites have created a "culture" which is sustained despite staff turnover. Such a culture seems to be accomplished by reaching a critical mass of individuals who regularly use the system and who promote its on-going use. This phenomenon may be particularly important for some applications where there is a lead time before the application has perceivable clinical benefit. For example, entering progress notes initially may take slightly longer than writing in the chart, especially if a terminal is not available on the clinician's desk at the time the patient is seen. The benefit for entering the note may not be readily apparent to the user as they enter those first notes. However, after three to five months of data entry, as the clinician starts to see the same patients again, often without a chart, the added benefit of entering the computer note so that it is readily retrievable becomes more and more apparent to the user. The phenomenon of a computer-oriented culture may be a critical one over a period of time in facilitating the continued use of clinical software at most facilities.

SOFTWARE FACTORS

Software factors include both general and specific components. Data retrieval applications appear to be more readily acceptable to clinicians than data entry applications. Local flexibility is important in tailoring both the input and the output to reflect the specific clinical setting in which they are being used. This local flexibility appears to be a U-shaped curve. If there is too much flexibility resulting in a complicated set-up, then this flexibility becomes more of a barrier than a facilitating factor. The software must fit the way that the user thinks and not try and force the user to learn a new way of either interacting with the patient or of conceptualizing the patient. In addition to fitting the way the user thinks, this software must have utility for the user.

The issue of time is also an important factor. In general, the use of the computer must take less time than the manual method unless the perceived benefit from using the computer software outweighs the added time from the users perspective. A simple application has a much higher chance of gaining acceptance than a complicated application. Complexity kills interest. Thus for data entry applications, interest decreases rapidly as the volume of data entry increases.

Specific software factors relate to the individual applications. One of the major factors that appears to differentiate between the successful and unsuccessful applications is the avoidance of duplication through the use of the software. For data entry, the computer should provide an output that replaces other work that the clinician would otherwise be doing. If this is not done, then a big administrative stick will be required to keep clinicians using the application. When the VA policy is approved for electronic signature of progress notes and other clinical entries, further acceptance of data entry among clinicians is anticipated. An electronic signature, which is affixed to the entered data by entering a third secret code, serves to be the legal equivalent of the hand-written signature and will preclude the need for having to manually sign the material after it has been printed out.

As more clinicians become computer literate the usual anxiety among clinicians may decrease, and more widespread use of the software may occur. For the VA this is a mixed blessing. People are becoming used to microcomputers that provide a very different interface than the VA's twelve year old system. They are becoming "spoiled" by the rapid response time of a dedicated computer system. This could actually discourage clinicians use of the "primitive" VA system, although it represents one of the more advanced clinically-oriented systems available in multiple facilities. However, there are plans to continue to develop and enhance the DHCP system to incorporate these new technologies, thus preventing such a backlash.

FUTURE APPLICATIONS

A number of new applications are planned for the MHS. These include a Clozapine monitoring system and the development of a mental health treatment plan. A decision support system for patients treated with neuroleptic has already been developed and is being systematically evaluated within the VA's DHCP system.

One of the strengths of operating within the DHCP environment is that many new applications are being developed for disciplines outside of mental health. These provide additional functions to mental health clinicians and may further enhance the clinical utility of the DHCP system. This benefit occurs even though the software is not specifically tailored for use just in mental health settings. As our colleagues and other disciplines develop new software, we are all able to benefit. For example, already in development or in testing are new applications including Order Entry by clinicians and the Problem Index, a history and physical examination, and on-line drug information system. The problem index is an enhanced Problem List with easier data entry for clinicians and with output formats that replace the Problem List in the medical records. A History and Physical Exam application is also in the planning stages that allows for entry of additional detail by specialists when doing a physical exam but requires only a simple organ system examination by non-specialists. Another interesting application current being tested at several VAs is an on-line pharmacy information system. Up-to-date drug interaction and side effect information can be looked up immediately from any terminal in the hospital.

These new applications will continue to extend the tools and resources available to clinicians who have the VA's DHCP system available to them. These applications complement those that are already in place and are designed to avoid the pitfalls that slowed down or prevented previous applications from being incorporated into daily clinical care.

The VA's DHCP system represents an interesting and potentially valuable chapter in the development of clinical software. Of particular importance is the fact that this software is designed to be used in multiple facilities and is evolving to provide clinicians with the ability to tailor the software to their own preferences. As the MHS becomes implemented at those VA sites now receiving additional hardware, we will continue to gain further understanding on the factors that lead to successful clinical applications being incorporated into clinical care. Inhibitory factors are also becoming more evident. These lessons will be used in the design of the next generation of clinical software both in mental health and in interdisciplinary applications.

REFERENCES

American Psychiatric Association. (1969). Computers in psychiatry. American Journal of Psychiatry, 125(1, Suppl.).

Glueck, B. D. (1974). Computers at the Institute of Living. In Crawford, J. L., Morgan, D. W., & Gianturco D. T. (Eds.), Progress in mental health information systems: Computer applications. Cambridge, MA: Ballinger.

Greist, J. H., & Klein, M. H. (1981). Computers in psychiatry. In Arieti, S. & Brodie, K.H. (Ed.), American handbook of psychiatry: Advances and new directions (Vol. 7, 2nd ed.). New York: Basic Books.

Hedlund, J. L., Vieweg, B. W., Wood, J. B., Cho, D. W., Evenson, R. C., Hickman, C. V., & Holland, R. A. (1981). Computers in mental health: A review and annotated bibliography (DHHS Publication No. ADM 81-1090). Washington, DC: U.S. Government Printing Office.

Johnson, J. H., & Williams, T. A. (1975). The use of on-line computer technology in a mental health admitting system. American Psychologist, 30, 388-390.

Laska, E. M. (1976). The Multi-State Information System for psychiatric patients. Medical Care, 14 (5, Suppl.), 223-229.

Lieff, J. L. (1987). Computer applications in psychiatry. Washington, DC: American Psychiatric Press.

McDonald, C. J., Sui, S. L., Smith, D. M., Tierney, W. M., Cohen, S. J., Weinberger, M., & McCabe, G. P. (1984). Reminders to physicians from an introspective computer medical record. Annals of Internal Medicine, 100, 130-138.

Schwartz, M. D. (Ed.). (1984). Using computers in clinical practice. New York: The Haworth Press, Inc.

Sidowski, J. B., Johnson, J. H., & Williams, T. A. (1980). Technology in mental health care delivery systems. Norwood, NJ: Ablex Publishing.

Obtaining Mental Health Software
by Telephone
from a Computerized
Bulletin Board System

Marvin J. Miller

KEYWORDS. Mental health software, telecommunications, computer bulletin boards, computerized patient testing

INTRODUCTION

One important aspect of the computer revolution has been the ability to send messages and computer files by telephone to another computer. This chapter will be a discussion of free standing computer Bulletin Board Systems (BBSs) but will also discuss other telecommunications services of interest to the mental health professional.

The telecommunications opportunities in today's market are wonderfully diverse and useful in a variety of different ways. Electronic mail can be sent to the opposite side of the globe at little or no cost. A chapter for a book can be transmitted in compact form across the country in one minute, edited and returned with comments within the hour. A discussion of the latest side-effects from a new psychotropic medication can be held on-line (simultaneously or over a period of hours) and the entire discussion be available in written format for all of the participants. A patient can be tested at a local doctor's office via phone line and the results printed out at the

Marvin J. Miller, MD, is Assistant Professor of Psychiatry at Indiana University School of Medicine and a staff psychiatrist at Larue Carter Hospital, 1315 W. Tenth Street, Indianapolis, IN 46202.

local office within minutes after the end of testing. A search of the relevant literature published over the last 20 years can be performed in several minutes with a print out of professional articles which might be relevant. A local physician's office can generate the day's billings and transmit them to local insurance companies over the phone line for more rapid payment. All the above are examples of a mental health professional using a computer and a phone line to get work done more quickly. One clinician can dial into the computer of a colleague across town or across the state and view the exact same information on his computer screen as that being viewed by a colleague. This can form the basis of a consultation or collaboration very nicely.

A computer bulletin board serves a more narrow subset of the above functions (Schwartz, 1985). It mainly exists for message exchange and for file transfer. Over 400 medical bulletin boards existed in the United States in 1991 and about 10 of these (Appendix I) focus primarily on the mental health field. In addition there are about 30 additional BBSs devoted to the lay audience wherein they exchange questions and ideas about various illnesses or treatment approaches.

LARGE COMMUNICATIONS NETWORKS

The free-standing BBS is only one component of a large network of communications systems which have served the computer community for over 20 years (Rickard, 1990). One of the oldest of these was funded by the military initially and served as a backbone of a national communications systems for a considerable time. The Defense Department system was called ARPANET and served as a way to link and convey messages between many different computer systems in industry and academia throughout the country. The philosophy and the software behind this effort were translated for the larger civilian community in a network called INTERNET/BITNET.[1] This system currently handles tens of thousands of E-Mail (electronic mail) messages each day. The messages are currently collected on a local system throughout the day and then transmitted at night at high speed under lower telephone rates to the intended destination. These messages may be routed through several systems before reaching their final address point. The system is so efficient that the messages cost only pennies to transmit and the costs are typically borne by universities and industries tied into the network. ARPANET will possibly be phased out over the next several years but the INTERNET/BITNET Communications System will likely continue to exist. There are periodic squabbles about the rather loose system of funding the network but this has proved adequate to this point.

Two large communications networks (Appendix II) devoted to the general public but containing some items of information relevant to the medical field are currently offered. CompuServe is available by subscription with an additional fee for connect time. It offers a wide variety of services (Green, 1985) but includes one particular discussion section/file section called Medsig. This is a forum for discussion among medical professionals regarding current issues. There are also hundreds of files available for downloading which have some applicability to the practice of medicine in general and to the mental health field in particular.

A newer communications service is offered jointly by IBM and Sears. This service is called Prodigy and offers an unlimited connect time for a fixed monthly fee. A limited number of messages can be exchanged as a part of the base fee with additional charges for extra messages which are exchanged.

The American Medical Association offered a communications network with a variety of services specifically for the physician community (AMANET). It included the ability to obtain continuing medical education credit over the phone, do literature searches and obtain full text copies of the articles, do a differential diagnosis of a difficult clinical situation, and exchange messages. This service however discontinued operations during 1990 because of low usage patterns. Interestingly the only replacement for this large multimillion dollar network was a small free standing bulletin board system called FedNet which is available to AMA members and to subscribing specialty organizations.

THE FREE STANDING BBS

The minimum equipment required to set up a free standing BBS is a computer, modem, and bulletin board system software. The configurations listed in Figure 1 demonstrate the variety of costs for an initial BBS. The minimal system would have to be dedicated to the single task of running the BBS. The recommended system would cost more but could run the BBS in background while being available as a regular computer for other tasks all the time. Monthly operating costs consist of less than $1.00 per day for the telephone line and whatever costs are necessary to maintain the computer equipment.

Hard Disk Size

An introductory system focused on the need to a very small select group of users might be able to get by with 20 megabytes of hard disk storage. This would be sufficient for up to 500 or so different computer files or up to several thousand messages. The larger BBSs today have 3-5 gigabytes of storage available. This could mean over 100,000 different computer programs available for downloading. The need for large capacity storage devices has made it increasingly popular to use optical disk storage systems for this purpose.

Modems

The modem translates the computer signals for transmission over the phone line. The current most popular speed for modem transmission is 2400 baud. Many BBSs however permit speeds as slow as 1200 baud or as fast as 9600 baud. The newest standards of compatibility for modems require the V.32 protocol for high speed data transmission and usually include the MNP as well as the V.42 protocols for error correction and data compression. By sending the data in more compact form the effective speed of data transmission over the phone line can be increased by 3-5 fold. Error correction insures that each character or command sent over the phone line is received error free or retransmitted until it can be received properly. There have been numerous software provisions for error free transmission of computer files (i.e., XMODEM) but the last several

Figure 1 - Sample BBS Configurations			
Minimal Configuration		Recommended Configuration	
386SX - 16MHz, VGA Color, 40 Meg Hard Disk, 1 Meg RAM	$899	386DX - 33MHz, 32K Cache, 120 Meg Hard Disk, VGA Color, 4 Meg Ram	$1899
2400 Baud Modem	$99	2400 Baud Modem	$99
Panasonic Printer KXP1123	$209	Panasonic Printer KXP1123	$209
Total	$1207		$2207

years have witnessed hardware methods for insuring data transmission over noisy phone lines. The older protocol which must be included in any modem compatibility list is the Hayes protocol. This standardizes a series of commands used in software addressing of the modem. Cost for a simple 2400 baud modem can be as little as $50 while a fully featured modem including all of the items mentioned above is $600-$700.

BBS Software

The oldest of the BBS software packages with a wide acceptance was the RBBS package (Remote Bulletin Board System). This software was produced by the Washington D.C. area personal computer club and for many years was the predominant system available across the country. It is still widely supported and recently received a prestigious "Editor's Choice" designation from PC Magazine (Salem, 1991). The current package in broadest use is called PC Board. Another package in widespread use is the Wildcat System. Both of these allow multiple phone lines coming into the same piece of software. There are a variety of sponsorship arrangements for a BBS. Some systems charge a flat annual fee (typically $25-$50) and grant use for a period of one year for a fixed number of minutes per day under that fee. A few charge fees based on the exact time of usage. There are a number of medical BBSs now sponsored by their professional societies (Neiburg, 1988) although none of these currently exist in the field of mental health. A variety of BBSs are simply sponsored by their operator and exist as a hobby (generally less expensive than golf or bowling). Many professional software companies maintain a BBS to disseminate information about their newest software products and to offer free or low cost upgrades to existing products. The amount of time required to operate a BBS varies greatly. The SYSOP (system operator) might devote as little as one hour per week for a low use system while the more popular multi-line systems may require one or two people full time to manage the system. SYSOP tasks include responding to messages on the system and checking incoming software and assigning it to particular usage areas.

Many persons are concerned about the possibility of viruses contained in software passing through a BBS. There are currently virus checking programs in existence and the potential for contamination from such a virus is very low if users practice reasonable precautions in checking new software for viruses.

SAMPLE BBS SESSION

The best way to illustrate the various features and potential offered in a BBS is to examine a sample BBS session. An example of this is enclosed in Appendix III. User responses are underlined. The first attempt to call a new BBS is complicated by the need to register in the new system. This includes giving some information about the location, phone number, type of system one is using and a few characteristic of the system. The registration generally takes one to two minutes and then one can explore the rest of the BBS.

Some BBSs insist on a call back for verification process. They will ask you to indicate a number at which your computer can be reached. The remote BBS calls back to see that a computer actually exists at that location in order to verify that this individual is real and has a specific phone number. This provides some additional safety for the BBS in attempting to verify the identity and location of the users.

After signing on the BBS it is customary to check for messages. The BBS will usually report if a personal message is awaiting a user. One can read the messages and respond to them or simply delete messages after they have been read. The message may have been left by someone on the local BBS or it may have been conveyed across country by one of the messages relay systems (Brunk, 1991). The oldest of these networks is FidoNet. This is a worldwide network of approximately 9,000 BBSs. A message on any of these connected systems will be automatically routed to the proper local BBS to be read by the intended recipient.

The most exciting part of a bulletin board system remains the ability to upload or download a piece of computer software. An illustration of downloading (having a remote computer send a piece of software to your own computer system) is included in the appendix. There are four main steps in this downloading process. In the example shown the letter D alerts the BBS of the desire to download. The BBS then requests the specific name of the piece of software to download. It then checks to see whether the user has clearance to download the software and whether there is sufficient remaining time to complete the download. If both of these conditions are favorable it then tells the user the estimated time for the download and tells the user to proceed with the download. The BBS system then waits for further commands from the user. At this point the user needs to send a command to initiate the download. The user must also indicate the file transfer routine being used. The oldest and still one of the most reliable methods for doing this is called XMODEM. It sends small packets of programs and checks for errors before sending the next packet. Software downloaded in this fashion is almost always received in good condition and usable immediately after the completion of the transfer. This holds true even when considering noisy phone lines. The software retransmits packets that were contaminated by a noisy phone line until a perfect transmission occurs. After giving the instruction for the transfer the remainder of the process is essentially automatic. Often the local communications program will keep track of the progress in the transfer and will update this continuously. At the end of the transfer there will be a message indicating it is completed. The BBS system will wait up to two minutes or so for further instructions from the user. If no further instructions are received the BBS will usually disconnect the two computers so that a new user may sign in. If the BBS does not provide for an automatic disconnect the user must initiate the disconnect by giving the good-bye command or the appropriate equivalent for that system. Failure to properly disconnect may result in a lengthy long distance phone bill for the user.

Some BBSs have the capability of running "doors." These allow a user to exit the BBS software and to participate in stand alone programs on the BBS computer. These might consist of a computer chess game being played by two individuals from different parts of the country. It might involve doing particular test scoring or various other software packages. After finishing a stand alone package the user exits back to the bulletin board and then exits from the total system.

Even though there are 8 or 10 different computer BBS software packages they have enough similarities so that it is quite simple to use a new BBS if a user has some familiar with the previous one.

A variety of common problems are encountered by the user of a BBS. The most frequent problem is the presence of telephone line noise. This becomes apparent to the user by the presence of various strange characters which suddenly appear on the computer screen and do not seem to have any connection with the message or words being exchanged. One step in eliminating this noise is to locate one's personal computer and modem at some distance from any television or appliance containing a large motor. If this is impossible or does not succeed in eliminating the noise there are additional steps available. One can purchase a radio frequency interference filter (RFI) in an electronic store or a telephone store for about $10.00. After plugging this into the phone line this will often screen out extraneous noise. Occasionally one must trace the course of a telephone line throughout the house or the office to see that it does not directly overlap a power line. If this kind of overlap is noticed it is wise to separate the two lines by 6 inches or more and the problem is helped considerably.

Philosophy of Shareware Computer Software

Bulletin boards would not experience their current popularity unless there was a wealth of software available to exchange through these channels. Software exchange on BBSs occurs under the principal that much software can be exchanged at no cost and some software can be exchanged on the honor system with the provision that the user return a small fee to the author in return for the privilege of using the software.

There are four main varieties of computer software available on bulletin boards. Public domain software has no copyright provisions and has been donated to the general public for use by anyone who pleases. There are usually few or no restrictions on its use. Freeware often contains a copyright notice but also contains the provision that this package is to be distributed at no cost and no one else distributing it may charge a fee except a nominal fee for copying and distributing disks containing the software. Authors may decide to retain copyright and label their software as freeware so that they can make further decisions at a later time regarding the possible commercial use of the software. The most common designation of software on a BBS is the label of "Shareware." This software carries copyright restriction and a provision that a user may have limited access to the software after which the user must pay a small designated fee. This process is often called registration and after paying this fee and registering the software there are sometimes limited additional materials or upgrades which are mailed to the user. This process depends on the honor system to provide income for the program author and yet some authors are able to achieve a very lucrative income through the process. Marketing and distribution costs under the shareware system are extremely low and the majority of the income can be allocated to the program authors.

A final form of software is sometimes available on systems. This is known as a demonstration program and contains most features of the actual commercial program but is limited by time or by capacity so that it is not very useful to the recipient. It does however demonstrate the main capabilities of the system and is distributed so that the users will buy the commercial product. Most BBS operators do not permit the presence of demonstration software on their system unless it delivers significant utility by itself.

Several areas of common courtesies need to be noted regarding the sharing of computer software on BBS's. It is very rude and usually illegal to modify software and claim it as the work of a new person. When registering a piece of software please respect the conditions of that registration. Also respect the telephone support conditions outlined in the agreement. If the software is distributed at no charge please don't expect free telephone support for the product. Arrange for a consulting fee if you really need support in such circumstances. Acknowledge the work of the software author in your use of the package and in any publications. Finally, and most importantly, upload software to the BBS occasionally if you expect the BBS to thrive! Don't just take but give something back to the fellow BBS users.

LEGAL ASPECTS OF BBSs

The presence of thousands of BBSs in this country pose a whole series of new legal questions. A recent discussion of this problem (Rose, 1991) outlines over 10 categories of laws which affect the operation of a bulletin board. It is clearly obvious that commercial programs which are not marketed under the shareware principal would not be allowed or distributed on a BBS. There are many questions regarding privacy issues of a BBS, contract law, financial law, securities laws and even educational laws that can be affected according to ways in which particular BBSs are used.

Computer programs which are produced directly as a result of a federal grant are in a gray area of ownership. Often the author makes slight additional modifications after the end of the federal grant and markets the package as a commercial program. It does seem clear that if the tax payers have paid for specific work to be performed under a contract that the taxpayers should have the resultant product. In spite of this some commercial software companies have insisted that the public has no rights to the program developed under a federal grant. There are different standards for grants administered under the small business program. This does allow for some specific ownership of product after the period of the grant. Most grants however administered by the National Institutes of Health or the National Institute of Mental Health do not specifically convey ownership to the recipient of that grant.

ENCOURAGING DEVELOPMENT OF SHAREWARE BY MENTAL HEALTH PROFESSIONALS

There has been an explosion of software available on BBSs for the general public. There are however less than a hundred programs specifically of interest to the mental health community which are available on BBSs. Various factors will need to change in order to encourage more development. The clarification of policy on software developed under federal grants could make a large change in the amount of software generally available. Professional societies need to take a hand in evaluating the quality of software available so that members can gain some confidence in specific packages. Professional societies may also wish to underwrite the development of certain packages and then make these available in a general fashion. Mental health professionals who use shareware packages from a BBS should be careful to honor the payment provisions of that package in order to foster further development. The sponsorship of a BBS should be considered by professional journals since they have a logical common interest in promoting the spread of technical and professional information in the field. Universities also need to take the lead in finding ways to recognize software authors. At the present time many schools have no mechanism to give academic or scholarly credit for a computer program. It lies somewhere between an article for a professional journal and an invention. A computer program allows the knowledge and expertise of a scholar to be disseminated and exercised over a lengthy period of time. This capability needs ways to be acknowledged in the academic circles.

SUMMARY

Telecommunications is an area developing a large and growing audience of users. The variety of functions available currently is great enough to merit serious consideration by any mental health professional. Exchange of computer software for the mental health professional via the phone line is a rapid and inexpensive way to disseminate programs.

NOTE

1. All trademarks referenced are the property of their respective companies.

REFERENCES

Brunk, M., (1991), An Introduction to Relaynet International Message Exchange, BBS Callers Digest, 2(7), 34-35.

Green, R., (1985), Using Compuserve as a Forum for Developing Applications Software, Computers in Psychiatry/Psychology, 7(2), 19-25.

Rickard, J., (1990), Internet Linking Up to the E-Mail World, Boardwatch Magazine, 4(7), 24-26.

Rose, L., (1991), Cyberspace and the Legal Matrix: Laws or Confusion, Boardwatch Magazine, 5(6), 27-32.

Salem, J., (1991), BBS Software, PC Magazine, 10(15), 231-300.

Schwartz, M., (1985), Network: Telecommunication, Computers in Psychiatry/Psychology, 7(4), 1-4

APPENDIX I

Mental Health Related BBSs

Maple Shade Opus – 609-482-8604 300/1200/2400 8N1.

Some software. Mainly discussion areas (i.e., hospice, recovery, 12 steps, caregivers)

PI Net 512-523-0236 300/1200 8N1

Both software and message areas. Large volume of callers. Mainly for Apple computer users.

Compsych – 518-564-3372 300/1200 8N1

Catalog of computer software from various manufacturers and bulletin areas. No software.

Social Work BBS – 906-774-8555 300-1200 8N1

New BBS. Both software and message areas.

Central Florida Psychology Forum BBS – 407-645-1658 8N1

Mostly for lay audience. Various message areas and some software.

Shrink Tank — 408-257-8131 300/1200/2400 8N1

Both software and message areas. Large volume of callers. Both for professionals and general public.

The Testing Station — 317-846-8917 300/1200/2400 8N1

Mainly software for mental health professionals. Sysop — Marvin Miller, M.D.

Psychology Forum — 214-368-5474 300/1200/2400 8N1

Both software and message areas. Both for general public and professionals.

UND Psych BBS — 701-777-4495 300/1200/2400 8N1

Mainly for psychology department of UND but some other users. Has message area and some software.

CSR Net (Community Support Network) — 617-353-5377 1200/2400 8N1

Funded by NIMH through the Community Support Program. Message area and some software.

Recently deceased BBSs:
Psych Forum — MSU,
American Psychological Association BBS
American Psych Exchange — (NY)

APPENDIX II

Products and Services Referenced in the Chapter

AMIA-The American Medical Informatics Association

AMIA is a professional organization dedicated to the development and application of medical informatics in the support of patient care, teaching, research, and health care administration. In 1991 AMIA became a full-time professional association with offices and staff of its own (formerly they had been managed by an association management company). This move is expected to result in improved services and development of new services to match the needs of its growing membership.

AMIA incorporates three formerly independent groups:

> AAMSI—the American Association of Medical Systems and Informatics
>
> SCAMC—the Board of Directors which operates the annual symposium on Computer Applications in Medical Care
>
> ACMI—the American College of Medical Informatics

For more information, contact:

> AMIA
> 4915 St. Elmo Ave.
> Suite 302
> Bethesda, MD 20814
> 301-657-1291

Bitnet/Internet Discussion Areas

BITNIS (BITNET-NLM Interconnection System)
Medical Telecommunication Networks (mailing list MEDNETS)
Psychology Newsletter (PSYCH)

Compuserve

Starter kits for CompuServe are available at most computer or software stores, or you can contact CompuServe at:

> CompuServe Customer Service
>   Administration Dept.
> P.O. Box 20212
> Columbus, OH 43220
> 800-848-8199

Computer Use in Social Services Network (CUSSN)

CUSSN is a network of human service professionals interested in using computers and other technologies in their practice. The three most important ventures are the CUSSN Newsletter, a network of computer BBSs called CUSSNET and a demo/shareware/freeware Disk Copy Service with a catalogue of available software. For more information contact: Dick Schoech, CUSS Network Coordinator, Associate Professor, University of Texas at Arlington, Box 19129, Arlington, TX 76019. (817) 273-3964.

BBS Nodes Carrying the CUSSNet Conference

Net/Node	BBS Name	City & State	Phone
10/300	Bruce's_Board	Barstow, CA	619-252-5150
11-301	Fido-Racer	Murray, KY	502-762-3140
104/52	Nurse_Link	Denver, CO	303-270-4936
104/62	Nojave Net	Westminster, CO	303-426-0623
105/10	Atarian_BBS	Portland, OR	503-245-9730
106/5433	TreeShare Genealogical BBS	Houston, TX	713-342-1174
109/507	Hd. Start RC	College Park, MD	301-985-7936
114/15	St_Joes_Hospital	Phoenix, AZ	602-235-9653
124/2121	Psychology Forum BBS	Dallas, TX	214-368-5474
129/75	Ecclesia_Place	Monroeville, PA	412-373-8612
130/10	DD_Connection	Arlington, TX	817-640-7880
132/111	On_Line_NH	Concord, NH	603-225-7161
134/202	Welcome to my nightmare	Sylvan Lake, AB, Canada	403-887-4514
138/115	Amocat BBS	Tacoma, WA	206-566-1155
138/116	Group Medical BBS	Tacoma, WA	206-582-3212
141/420	The Handicap News	Shelton, CT	203-337-1607
150/101	Black_Bag_BBS	Newark, DE	302-731-1998
157/3	Nerd's Nook	Rocky River, OH	216-356-1431
202/606	Hillcrest BBS	San Diego, CA	619-291-0544
203/11	The Broken Rose	Sacramento, CA	916-483-8624
203/454	Sacramento Peach Child	Sacramento, CA	916-451-0225
205/80	TOTTBBS	Fresno, CA	209-292-6403
208/200	Software Silo	Stockton, CA	209-477-9502
265/102	Connect! BBS	Dale City, VA	703-670-5037
266/12	Maple_shade_Opus	Maple Shade, NJ	609-482-8604
267/41	The_Host_BBS	Glens Falls, NY	518-793-9574
275/429	HandiNet BBS	Virginia Beach, VA	804-496-3320
300/7	First_Dibs	Tucson, AZ	602-881-8720
305/101	NASW_New_Mexico	Las_Cruces, NM	505-646-2868
321/109	Pioneer_Val_PCUGI	Amherst, MA	413-256-1037
321/203	VETLink#1	Pittsfield, MA	413-443-6313
343/35	HDS_Univ_of_Wash	Seattle, WA	202-543-3719
381/5	Micro Applications	El Paso, TX	915-591-1090
382/1	Capitol City	Lake Travis, TX	512-335-7949
382/5	Health-Link	Austin, TX	512-444-9908
387/404	ACS_People_Connection	San Antonio, TX	512-647-8189
254/11	Polynet	London, UK	441-580-1690
2:253/151	TOPPSI	Dublin, Ireland	353-1-7110
2:253/152	UK_Healthlink	Wigan, UK	44-942-722984
2:256/97	LogOn-On-Tynedale	Hexham, UK	44-434606639
2:273/105	Datawerken_IT	Remmerden, Holland	318376-15363
2:331/201	Amigaline	Bologna, Italy	31-1810-15600
2:512/120	STEBIS	Leiden, Holland	31-71-320002
2:7105/10	Waco Host	Utrecht, Holland	31-3438-21410
3:634/388	Axiom BBS	Melbourne, Australia	61-3-509-4417

DIALOG Medical Connection

Medical Connection is the online medical information service of DIALOG Information Services. It provides a collection of online reference sources for biomedical researchers, physicians, and health professionals.

For more information about all DIALOG services, contact:

> DIALOG Marketing
> 800-334-2564
> 415-858-2700
> 3460 Hillview Ave.
> Palo Alto, CA 94304

FEDNET

FEDNET is now offered by the AMA Office of County/State Relations. It provides an online bulletin board for state, county and specialty medical societies, and includes the AMA Washington Report and information on other legislative and organizational activity of note. FEDNET is now a private information service available only to participating medical societies. For further information, contact:

> Gloria Green
> American Medical Association
> Office of County/State Relations
> 515 N. State St.
> Chicago, IL 60610

Fidonet Echos

Computer Users in the Social Sciences (CUSS)
Mental Health (MENTAL-HEALTH)

GRATEFUL MED

GRATEFUL MED is an easy-to-use, fill-in-the-blanks MEDLARS search assist software package developed by the National Library of Medicine. it is available for IBM-PCs and compatibles (DOS version), as well as in a Macintosh version. The price for either version is $29.95 plus $3.00 handling.

GRATEFUL MED must be ordered from the National Technical Information Service. The order number for the IBM-PC version is PB86-196083/

GBB. American Express, VISA, and MasterCard are accepted. Add a $7.50 billing fee if you are using a purchase order. GRATEFUL MED costs $29.95 plus $3.00 for handling. Order from:

U.S. Department of Commerce
National Technical Information Service
5285 Port Royal Road
Springfield, VA 22161
Phone: 703-487-4650
Or fax: 703-321-8547
(with credit card or PO information)

Medicine Conference on BIX, the BYTE Information Exchange

BIX is the online information service of BYTE magazine. It offers a number of online discussion areas of conferences, including one called "Medicine," for information on "computers in the medical and health services fields."

Within the Medicine conference there are discussion topics such as software, information systems, academia, education, medicine, and others.

Subscription information:

Subscription of BIX is available for a quarterly fee of $39. There are also connect charges (Tymnet) of $6 per hour in prime time (6 am to 7 pm, Monday through Friday) and $3 per hour in non-prime hours (all other hours, including weekends).

For more information or to subscribe, contact:

Byte Information Exchange
1 Phoenix Mill Lane
Peterboro, NH 03458
603-924-7681
800-227-2983

MEDICOM Drug Interaction System

Published by Professional Drug Systems, MEDICOM analyzes patient data for potential drug interactions between prescription and OTC drugs, drug-food or drug-nutrient interferences, and allergy and disease contraindications. It is currently available as a PC-based product. For further information, contact:

Amy DeWein
Professional Drug Systems
2388 Schuetz Rd.
St. Louis, MO 63146

MEDLINE (MEDlars onLINE)

MEDLINE is a database of biomedical information from 1966 to the present, gathered from approximately 3,500 U.S. and foreign journals. Updated weekly, it contains about six million citations in both current and archived files. Backfiles are grouped in two-year increments. The current 1989-91 file contains more than 635,000 entries as of January 1991.

For more information about MEDLINE and other NLM databases and services, call the MEDLARS Management Section of the National Library of Medicine at 301-496-6193.

PC Physician

PC Physician Medical Computing Resource Guide is a disk based collection of information about computerized tools available for the medical professional. Searches for particular information are very fast. It is updated every 6 months and is available for the IBM or Macintosh. For more information contact: PC Physician, 3300 Mitchell Lane, Suite 390, Boulder, CO 80301, (303) 443-8085 or (303) 443-7653 (Fax).

PsyComNet

PsyComNet is a telecommunications service for psychiatrists. Interactive conferencing, E-Mail, notice boards, and data libraries are available 24-hours a day on this service.

Notice boards are computerized bulletin boards where messages may be brought to the attention of others and messages left by others may be answered. Data libraries contain programs and textual material (such as bibliographies), that are available for downloading. PsyComNet notice boards and data libraries are devoted to the following topics:

— Psychotherapy/Psychoanalysis
— Psychopharmacology

— Neuropsychology
— Adult Disorders
— Child/Adolescent Disorders

For more information, contact:

Ivan K. Goldberg, M.D.
PsyComNet
1346 Lexington Ave.
New York, NY 10128
212-876-7800

PaperChase

PaperChase is one of the most popular and easy-to-use ways to access the MEDLINE data base. Developed at Boston's Beth Israel Hospital. Paper-Chase was designed specifically for use by health care professionals.

For more information, contact PaperChase at 350 Longwood Avenue, Boston, MA 02115, or call 800/722-2075 from U.S. and Canada (within Massachusetts, call 617/278-3900).

PsychINFO

PsychINFO is the online information service of the American Psychological Association. It is available online through BRS, DIALOG, and Compuserve.

PsychINFO
information, contact:

PsychINFO User Services
1400 North Uhle Street
Arlington, VA 22201
800-336-4890
703-247-7829 (in VA)

UUNET Technologies, Inc.

UUNET Technologies provides access to USENET news, UUCP mail, Unix source archives, and many standards (including the Internet RFCs and comp.std.unix archives).

For more information, contact:

UUNET Technologies, Inc.
3110 Fairview Park Dr.
Suite 570
Falls Church, VA 22042
703-876-5050 (voice)
FAX: 703-876-5059

Appendix III
Sample BBS Session

After dialing in to the Testing Station BBS
the following interaction is a sample session
for an initial user.

THE TESTING

STATION

A BBS for psychiatrists and psychologists. If
you have not already done so please leave me a
message with the enter (E) command noting your
full address and telephone number.

Everyone please read Bulletin 7.
Read Bulletin 5 to learn about computer conference.

Marvin Miller, M.D., 8918 Coventry Rd.,
Indpls, IN 46260, (317) 8465688

What is your FIRST name? James
What is your LAST name? Smith
Checking Users...
User not found
Are you 'JAMES SMITH' ([Y],N)? y
What is your CITY and STATE? Indpls, IN
THE TESTING STATION

JAMES SMITH from INDPLS, IN
C)hange FIRST name/LAST name/CITY and STATE,
D)isconnect, [R]egister? R

Enter PASSWORD you'll use to logon again? ....
Re-Enter PASSWORD for Verification (Dots Echo)? ....
Please REMEMBER your password

CAN YOUR TERMINAL DISPLAY LOWER CASE ([Y]/N)? Y
UPPER CASE and lower

========== GRAPHICS OPTIONS =======================

<N>one - you can receive and display only the following
characters:
ABCDEFGHIJKLMNOPQRSTUVWXYZ   abcdefghijklmnopqrstuvwxyz
0123456789 and standard punctuation characters.

<A>scii - you can receive and display all 256 ascii codes
of the IBM PC character set such as the heart ^C and

straight line ——.

<C>olor - your communications package supports ANSI
screen commands
            (e.g. this blinks in green) as well as the
            music commands of BASIC

GRAPHICS for text files and menus
Change from N to N)one, A)scii-IBM, C)olor-IBM,
H)elp ([ENTER] quits)? n
Text GRAPHICS: None

Do you want COLORIZED prompts ([Y],N)? n
Highlighting Off

File transfer protocol: The method you want to
use to transfer files to RBBS-PC ("upload") or
to obtain files from RBBS-PC ("download").

TIPS:

1. You may want not to have a default transfer
protocol if you use a variety of protocols.
Select the N)one option and RBBS-PC will ask for your
preferred protocol before each file transfer.

2. The protocol you want RBBS-PC to use must also
be used by your communications package. Protocols
available in RBBS-PC include Ascii (no error
checking), Xmodem, Xmodem/CRC, and Ymodem.

Xmodem is the most widely supported, but Ymodem and
Zmodem are faster.

A)scii
C)rc Xmodem
K)ermit
X)modem
Y)modem (1K Xmodem)
W)indowed Xmodem
N)one - Cancel
Select Protocol? x
TurboKey: act on 1 character command without
waiting for [ENTER]
Want TurboKeys (Y/[N])? n
TurboKey Off

Appendix III (continued)

Your security level 5 indicates that you have the
minimum security necessary to log onto this board.
Logging JAMES SMITH
RBBS-PC CPC17.2B/0806 NODE 1, OPERATING AT 1200 BAUD,N,8,1

Welcome to THE TESTING STATION
Dedicated to the free exchange of information.

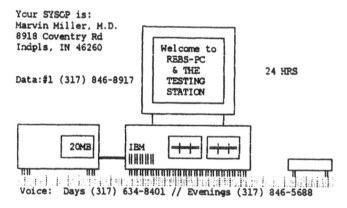

Your SYSOP is:
Marvin Miller, M.D.
8918 Coventry Rd
Indpls, IN 46260

Data:#1 (317) 846-8917

Welcome to
RBBS-PC
& THE
TESTING
STATION

24 HRS

20MB   IBM

Voice: Days (317) 634-8401 // Evenings (317) 846-5688

Number	Description	Revised
1.	Welcome To The Bulletin Board	05-25-89
2.	Listing of medical bulletin boards	05-26-89
3.	Explains file extensions	07-28-85
4.	Using this BBS	08-17-85
5.	News of Computers in Mental Health Mtg Coming up on April 19, 1991	01-16-91
6.	Other BBS's around the country	02-01-90
7.	Legal notice.	04-24-90

READ A BULLETIN BY GIVING # OF BULLETIN AND PRESSING ENTER
Read what bulletin(s), L)ist, N)ew ([ENTER] = none)? N

Checking messages in MAIN..
Sorry, JAMES, NO MAIL for you

RBBS-PC CPC17.2B/0806 Node 1

Caller # 115 # active msgs: 23 Next msg # 46

USERS: used 55 avl 431 MSGS: used 23 avl 77 MSG REC: used 176 avl 325
Upload disk has 991232 bytes free

```
71 min left
+-------------------------------+        +----------------------------------+
|          MESSAGES             |        |                                  |
| <C>omments to SYSOP           |        |      Sysop: Marvin Miller M.D.   |
| <E>nter message               |        |      Voice: 317 8465688          |
| <J>oin conf(Not active)       |        +----------------------------------+
| <K>ill message                |
| <Q>uick scan messages   +---------------------------+
| <P>ersonal mail         |                           |
| <R>ead messages         |         UTILITIES         +---------------------+
| <S>can messages         +---------------------------|      ELSEWHERE      |
|                         | <H>elp...Are you lost?     | <L>ines per page    |
| <O>perator chat         | <V>iew conf(Not active)    | <B>ulletins         |
|                         | <W>ho else (Not active)    | <D>oors (NOT OPEN)  |
|                         | <X>pert toggle ON/OFF      | <F>iles subsystem   |
+-------------------------| <?>Functions supported     | <G>oodbye           |
                          +---------------------------+ | <I>nitial welcome   |
                                                        | <U>tilities subsystem|
                                                        +---------------------+
```

MAIN command <?,A,B,C,D,E,F,H,I,J,K,O,P,Q,R,S,T,U,V,W,X>? r
Message base MAIN
Msg # 3-45 (H)elp,S)ince,L)ast, T)o, F)rom,M)ine, text, [Q]uit)?s
Msg #: *3
  From: GORDON FORBES   Sent: 01-20-91 22:37
    To: SYSOP   Rcvd: 01-21-91 07:48
    Re: COMMENT

I registered a couple of weeks ago. I got your number from ShrinkTank.
I was able to log on one time, but now I am not recognized. Am I doing
something wrong?

Gordon

More
[Y]es,N)o,C)ontinuous,A)bort,R)eply,T)hread,=)reread,+,-,K)ill?

                     Msg #: *5
  From: SYSOP   Sent: 01-23-91 14:34
    To: GORDON FORBES   Rcvd: 01-25-91 00:05
    Re: REGISTER

You're registered OK now. I installed new software.

                     Msg #: 1

  From: SYSOP   Sent: 04-15-91 08:03
    To: ALL   Rcvd: 04-16-91 01:58
    Re: WELCOME

Welcome to THE TESTING STATION BBS. If you have been on this BBS before
you will notice some changes. I have updated the BBS software so now
everyone will have to re-register. (You obviously have already done
this if you are reading this message.) Please use this BBS as it
benefits you. Upload software to keep the BBS going. Contributions

Appendix III (continued)

can be sent to Marvin Miller, M.D., 8918 Coventry, Indpls, IN 46260 and
will be used to help pay the phone costs. At present I pay most of
those myself. Voice phone lines are (317) 634-8401 #583 during the day
and (317) 846-5688 after 5 pm.

More [Y]es,N)o,C)ontinuous,A)bort,R)eply,T)hread,=)reread,+,-,K)ill?
  70 min left

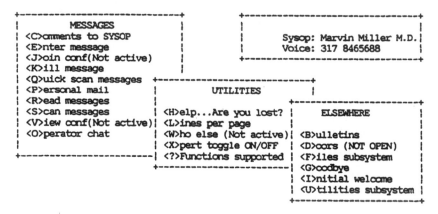

```
+-----------------------------+        +-----------------------------------+
|        MESSAGES             |        |                                   |
| <C>omments to SYSOP         |        |        Sysop: Marvin Miller M.D.  |
| <E>nter message             |        |        Voice: 317 8465688         |
| <J>oin conf(Not active)     |        +-----------------------------------+
| <K>ill message              |
| <Q>uick scan messages  +-----------------------------+
| <P>ersonal mail        |                             |
| <R>ead messages        |        UTILITIES            |
| <S>can messages        +-----------------------------+
| <V>iew conf(Not active)| <H>elp...Are you lost? |     ELSEWHERE
| <O>perator chat        | <L>ines per page      |
|                        | <W>ho else (Not active)| <B>ulletins
+------------------------| <X>pert toggle ON/OFF | <D>oors (NOT OPEN)
                         | <?>Functions supported| <F>iles subsystem
                         +-----------------------+ <G>oodbye
                                                   <I>nitial welcome
                                                   <U>tilities subsystem
                                                   +-------------------+
```

MAIN command <?,A,B,C,D,E,F,H,I,J,K,O,P,Q,R,S,T,U,V,W,X>? f

70 min left

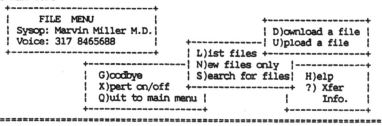

```
+-----------------------------+
|      FILE MENU              |        +--------------------+
| Sysop: Marvin Miller M.D.   |        | D)ownload a file   |
| Voice: 317 8465688          |  +-------------| U)pload a file      |
+-----------------------------+  | L)ist files +--------------------+
               +-------------------| N)ew files only |-------------+
               | G)oodbye          | S)earch for files| H)elp       |
               | X)pert on/off     +------------------+ ?) Xfer     |
               | Q)uit to main menu |                 | Info.       |
               +-------------------+                  +-------------+
```
===

FILE command <?,D,G,H,L,N,P,Q,S,U,V,X>? l

* Ctrl-K(^K) / ^X aborts. ^S suspends ^Q resumes *

CATEGORIES OF FILES AVAILABLE

1. Psych- Adults   7. Spreadsheets/Databases/Util
2. Psych- Children   8. Not used
3. Medical Education   9. Misc and text files
4. Other Medical Programs
5. Office manage/finances
6. Statistics

TO SEE THE FILES AVAILABLE IN A CATEGORY TYPE NUMBER
OF CATEGORY.
What directory(s) (U)pload,A)ll,L)ist,E)xtended +/-, [Q]uit)? 1

* Ctrl-K(^K) / ^X aborts. ^S suspends ^Q resumes *

                CLINICAL PROGRAMS

(For IBM and compatibles unless noted differently)

```
********************************************************
STRESSS.ZIP   117K    02-09-91  System to count and manage stress
CAS.ZIP       156k    01-22-91  Clinical Assessment System
SMOKERS.ZIP   57k     01-22-91  7 day plan to stop smoking
STRESS2.ZIP   36k     01-22-91  Eval symptoms of stress
WCST.ZIP      78k     12-13-90  Wisconsin Card Sorting Demo - Nice
LOVE.ZIP      13K     06-07-90  Evaluates 6 different styles of
                                interacting in a romantic relation-
                                ship.
SCL-45.ZIP    55k     04-26-89  Abbreviated version of SCL
                                Generates same scales
B_MOD_1.ZIP   209K    03-25-89  Teaches behavior mod concepts.
B_MOD_2.ZIP   90K     03-25-89  Needed with above.
DSM3R688.ZIP  120K    11-01-88  Diagnostic decision tree - for adults
More [Y]es,N)o,C)ontinuous,A)bort? n
What directory(s) (U)pload,A)ll,L)ist,E)xtended +/-, [Q]uit)?
```

    68 min left
    +-----------------------------+
    | FILE MENU | +--------------------+
    | Sysop: Marvin Miller M.D. | | D)ownload a file |
    | Voice: 317 8465688 | +----------| U)pload a file |
    +-----------------------------+ | L)ist files +------------------+
            +--------------------+----| N)ew files only |------------+
            | G)oodbye | S)earch for files| H)elp |
            | X)pert on/off   +------------------+ ?) Xfer |
            | Q)uit to main menu | | Info. |
            +--------------------+   +---------------------+
    ===

FILE command <?,D,G,H,L,N,P,Q,S,U,V,X>? d
Download what file(s)? wcst.zip
Searching for WCST.ZIP.

File Size   : 617 blocks 78976 bytes
Transfer Time: 14 min, 3 sec (approx)
Xmodem SEND of wcst.zip ready. <Ctrl X> aborts

(At this point the user gives the command to download the file. This
command on Qmodem is the PageDown key followed by the X key to choose
XMODEM)

Download successful

Appendix III (continued)

55 min left

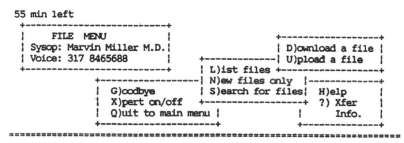

```
+--------------------------+
|      FILE MENU           |                  +------------------+
| Sysop: Marvin Miller M.D.|                  | D)ownload a file |
| Voice: 317 8465688       |    +-------------| U)pload a file   |
+--------------------------+    | L)ist files +------------------+
             +------------------| N)ew files only |-------------+
             | G)oodbye         | S)earch for files|  H)elp     |
             | X)pert on/off    +-----------------+  ?) Xfer    |
             | Q)uit to main menu |              |     Info.    |
             +--------------------+              +--------------+
```
==

FILE command <?,D,G,H,L,N,P,Q,S,U,V,X>?

FILE command <?,D,G,H,L,N,P,Q,S,U,V,X>? s
Search for (in file name/desc, wildcards name only, [ENTER] quits)? sc*.*

* Ctrl-K(^K) / ^X aborts. ^S suspends ^Q resumes *

CATEGORIES OF FILES AVAILABLE

1. Psych- Adults   7. Spreadsheets/Databases/Util
2. Psych- Children   8. FASTTEST Files
3. Medical Education   9. Misc and text files
4. Other Medical Programs
5. Office manage/finances
6. Statistics

54 min left

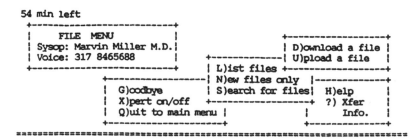

```
+--------------------------+
|      FILE MENU           |                  +------------------+
| Sysop: Marvin Miller M.D.|                  | D)ownload a file |
| Voice: 317 8465688       |    +-------------| U)pload a file   |
+--------------------------+    | L)ist files +------------------+
             +------------------| N)ew files only |-------------+
             | G)oodbye         | S)earch for files|  H)elp     |
             | X)pert on/off    +-----------------+  ?) Xfer    |
             | Q)uit to main menu |              |     Info.    |
             +--------------------+              +--------------+
```
==

FILE command <?,D,G,H,L,N,P,Q,S,U,V,X>? g
End session (Y,[N])? y

Now: 03-14-91 at 08:11:56
On for 21 mins, 5 secs
 54 min left for next call today
JAMES, Thanks and please call again!
iµ/ ⌐

The Development
of the Missouri Automated
Reinforcer Assessment (MARA):
An Update

Madeleine Vatterott
Jayne Callier
Matthew Hile

KEWORDS. Computerized patient testing, behavior therapy, mental health software, developmental disabilities software

SUMMARY. The Missouri Automated Reinforcer Assessment (or MARA) is a computer program developed to determine a collection of reinforcers for use in behavior programs, activity selection, and to provide general preference information. The goal of the Missouri Automated Reinforcer Assessment is to provide a thorough, yet efficient assessment of an individual's preferences via the computer, and to present the obtained information in a usable manner to a teacher, mental health professional, parent, caretaker, etc. The MARA was designed for verbal individuals who are most likely to be on a reinforcer program. These individuals include persons who are developmentally delayed, young children with behavior or motivation problems, adult and child psychiatric inpatients, and individuals who have suffered a brain trauma.

In this paper, a general discussion regarding reinforcers and reinforcer assessments will be presented, with a discussion of the advantages and disadvantages of an automated assessment. After this background information, the procedure used to obtain the items in

Madeleine Vatterott is in private practice. The work reported here was completed while Dr. Vatterott was a post doctoral fellow at the Missouri Institute of Mental Health. Address correspondence to Madeleine Vatterott, (MARA), Missouri Institute of Mental Health, 5247 Fyler, St Louis, MO 63139.

the program will be presented, followed by a description of the automated program.

REINFORCERS AND REINFORCER ASSESSMENTS

Positive reinforcers are often used in behavioral treatment for the acceleration of adaptive behavior and deceleration of maladaptive behavior. A positive reinforcer is typically defined by its effect on behavior — if "x" applied following a behavior increases the likelihood of that behavior in the future, "x" is a reinforcer. Ideally, in selecting a reinforcer to use in treatment, each potential reinforcer should be tested for its effect on behavior. Unfortunately, the amount of time necessary to assess systematically each reinforcer limits the usefulness of this procedure in most situations. Other ways of assessing reinforcer preferences include observing what the individual typically does in a free situation, providing the individual with samples of each reinforcer or a list of potential reinforcers and then asking them to choose their favorite, and simply asking them what they like (Heron, 1987).

There are many paper and pencil assessments of reinforcer preferences available in the literature (see Table 1). Although these assessments are useful in determining an individual's preferences, many of them are too brief to obtain very specific preferences or too lengthy and time-consuming to answer. In addition, information regarding how much more a person would like to receive a particular reinforcer seems pertinent to obtain, given that what they chose may be used in a reinforcer program.

ADVANTAGES AND DISADVANTAGES OF AN AUTOMATED ASSESSMENT

An automated assessment may increase the efficiency of a reinforcer assessment because the questions presented are tailored to the individual's responses. For example, if a subject indicated that he or she did not like sports, the assessment would not ask them about their preference for specific sports. An automated assessment also speeds scoring and reporting time over paper and pencil surveys.

By using a computer, an individual's reported level of satiation

Table 1. List of Previous Paper and Pencil Reinforcer

         Assessments

The Reinforcement Survey Schedule (Cautela & Kastenbaum, 1967)

Modified Reward Preference Assessment Procedure (Cartwright & Cartwright,

1970)

Survey Schedule of Rewards for Children (Keat, 1974)

The Children's Reinforcement Survey Schedule (Phillips

Fischer, & Singh, 1977)

The Children's Reinforcement Survey Schedule (Cautela & Brion-Meisels, 1979)

The Reinforcement Survey Schedule for Special Needs Children (Dewhurst &

Cautela, 1980)

How to Select Reinforcers (Hall & Hall, 1980)

The Autism Reinforcer Checklist for Children (Atkinson, Jenson, Rovner,

Cameron, Van Wagenen, & Petersen, 1984)

Motivation Assessment Scale (Durand & Crimmins, 1986)

The Reinforcement Inventory (Willis & LaVigna, 1987)

The Reinforcer Responsiveness Checklist (Bihm, 1989)

or deprivation for a preferred reinforcer could be easily assessed. For example, only for the items selected as preferred, there will be a question regarding how much more a person would like to have that item (ex., "How much more would you like hamburgers for dinner?"). The assumption of this line of questioning is that an item will be more reinforcing if a person indicates that they would like to have more often, than if the person states they have the item enough already. This assumption is an extrapolation of the Response Deprivation Hypothesis developed by Timberlake and Allison (1974), in which opportunities to perform responses that were kept below a normal steady state rate could be used as a reinforcer.

An automated assessment would allow the users to add easily items that are not on a given reinforcer list. These items could then be used for later comparison with other items that are already on a list. For example, if there is a question regarding a food preference, a user could select "other" and type in their response.

By automating the assessment, specific questions that are inappropriate for a younger age could easily be deleted. For example, if an individual's age is below 18, questions regarding alcohol consumption and physical intimacies could easily not be presented.

Some disadvantages of an automated assessment include the physical requirements of having a computer, and having the computer available to the individuals taking the assessment.

Another disadvantage is that some individuals may be intimidated by using a computer. In these cases, it may be necessary for the staff, etc., to give the person additional instruction, or enter the answers for them.

Finally, if a person is unfamiliar with a keyboard, and if they like many of the items presented, the MARA may actually take longer than a thorough paper and pencil assessment. This may not be a problem if there is time available, and the person enjoys taking the survey.

Item Collection

A pilot study was performed to obtain specific reinforcing items (appropriate for the targeted populations) to be included in the MARA program. Before conducting this study, specific information was not available regarding appropriate reinforcers for these groups.

An open-ended reinforcer survey covering a range of categories was given to the targeted populations. The general questions used in the survey were obtained from a review of previous surveys.

There were 45 individuals who participated from the following populations: two units from a state hospital—a brain trauma unit (n = 8), and a chronic schizophrenic unit (n = 11); an inpatient children's and adolescent psychiatric population (n = 8); and an institutional (n = 8) and community setting (n = 10) for individuals who are developmentally delayed. These participants were required to have receptive and expressive communication skills to respond to the examiner's questions. These individuals ranged in age from 8 to 64, with 8 of them under 21, 9 who were 21-30 years old, 11 who were 31-40, 9 of them were 41-50, and 8 participants were over 50 years of age. There were 28 males, and 17 females.

Signed consents were obtained from each participant, and from their guardian (if necessary).

The open-ended, paper and pencil questionnaire used to assess reinforcer preferences contained 30 questions covering 6 general reinforcer categories: food and drink, social interactions, general activities, solitary activities, tangibles, and "other." The questionnaire ranged in abstraction from "What do you most like to eat for dinner?" to "What do you like most?"

After the purpose of the study was explained, each participant was asked to give 3 responses to each of the 30 questions. The participants were sometimes asked to give more specific information if it was thought that this may be pertinent to the MARA program. For example, if the question was "What are your favorite things to drink?", and the subject responded with "Soda," he or she would be asked "Which kind of soda do you like best?"

The items obtained were scored for the frequency of occurrence across the different populations. The most frequently occurring responses are presented in Table 2. Approximately the 10 most frequent items were used in the MARA program.

In addition to providing the specific items to be used in MARA, the pilot study directed the wording of the questions to be asked in the MARA, and indicated some additional questions to ask. Some questions initially used in the paper and pencil questionnaire were simplified in the MARA. For example, the question "If you had 10 dollars to buy anything that you wanted, what things would you like to buy?" was reworded to "What would you buy if you had some money?"

THE MISSOURI AUTOMATED REINFORCER ASSESSMENT (MARA)

The MARA is an automated assessment that presents a question regarding a reinforcer, and a menu of specific responses. Based on an individual's response, the program proceeds to the next question. For example, if the subject selects the answer "Very Much" to the question "How much do you like snacks or desserts?", a list of specific snacks and desserts would be presented. If the subject

Table 2. Most Preferred Items from Open-ended Questionnaire*

Question	#1	#2	#3
1. Eat for dinner	chicken(17)**	steak/pizza/fish(9)	pork(8)***
2. Snacks	cake(14)	ice cream(12)	sandwich(8)
3. Drinks	soda(32)	fruit juice(16)	tea(13)
4. Indoor games	cards(26)	games(15)	indoorsports(9)
5. Pets/animals	dogs or puppies(28)	cats or kittens(25)	horse/bird(4)
6. To read	magazines(7)	books/fiction(6)	the Bible(5)
7. Topics to learn	school topics(21)	mechanics(5)	sports(3)
8. Type of music	rock and roll(16)	country(12)	classical(8)
9. Sport to play	baseball(22)	basketball(11)	none(8)
10. Sport to watch	baseball(25)	football(6)	basktball/ ice hockey(5)
11. Do outside	go for a walk(14)	sports(9)	yardwork(8)
12. Want to buy	eat or drink(21)	vehicle(13)	clothes(11)
13. Chores	housework(21)	none/get job(9)	run househld(5)
14. Reward self-day	a drink(19)	to eat(17)	watch TV/movie(5)
15. Do in free-time	watch TV(10)	music/sleep/read(8)	cards/?(4)****
16. Free-time, if anything	visit someone(14)	vacation(10)	I don't know(7)
17. Activity to try	skiing(6)	water sports/none(5)	ice-skating(4)
18. Enough attention	Yes (30)	No (11)	I don't know(3)
19. Type attention	individual/praise(7)	none(5)	?/touch(4)
20. One candy now or two later	one now (15)	two later (25)	I don't know(1)
21. Help someone do	housework(10)	school work(5)	feel better 5)
22. Extra good work	money(21)	food(8)	a gift(6)
23. Others do, say	say nice things(11)	?/nothing/visit(6)	give things(4)
24. With a friend	talk or visit(15)	out to eat(6)	to movie/bar(4)
25. With opp. sex	touch or sex(12)	talk or visit(9)	personal (7) characteristics
26. By yourself	read/TV or movies(9)	listen to music(7)	sleep(6)
27. In life	relationships/ job(5)	helping someone/ I don't know(4)	yardwork/ housework(4)
28. Like most	clothes/sports/ family(5)	opposite sex/friend /food(4)	music/ (3) I don't know
29. Three wishes	money(15)	car/motorcycle(10)	independence(9)
30. Anything else	nothing(7)	I don't know(4)	shop/TV/food(3)

* n = 45
** Number in parentheses indicates total frequency of occurrence
*** The symbol "/" is used when items occurred with the same frequency
**** The "?" is used as a short method for representing "I don't know"

had responded ''Not at all'' to the question, a new reinforcer question would be given.

The question progression follows the sequence of: a general reinforcer category question, a list of specific items in that general category, further item specification (if necessary), and a question regarding the level of satiation or deprivation for each item. A response is required for each question. Following the questions, a list of items is presented of items chosen from a particular category of reinforcers or that the subject indicated they want more of, and the user is then asked to select their favorites.

System requirements. This program was written in Knowledge Pro (copyright © 1987, Knowledge Garden Inc.), an expert system development shell. It does not require that the user own Knowledge Pro. It requires an IBM or IBM compatible computer. While it is usable with an 8088 microprocessor, practically speaking, at least a 286 microprocessor is required. It requires 640K RAM, and approximately 1MB free space on the hard drive. It can be used with monochrome or color monitors, with or without a mouse.

General categories. After obtaining some demographic information from the subject, general categories of reinforcers are presented on the screen and the user is asked to indicate if, or how much, they like that particular category. For example, the subject will be asked "Do you like to watch sports?" or "How much do you like desserts?"

Specific items. Based on an individual's response to the general question (i.e., if they said they liked it or they liked it "Very much" or "A little"), a menu of specific items from a category is then presented. The specific items presented from a category will be the most frequent answers obtained from the pilot study.

Individuals are then asked to select 3 of the items from the menu that they like best. For example, if a subject indicated that they like snacks or desserts ("Very Much" or "A Little"), he or she will be presented with a list of approximately 10 specific snacks or desserts (ex., ice cream, cookies, chips, cake, pie, etc.). If a particular specific item chosen requires even more detailed information (for example, flavor of ice cream), then a pop-up menu listing the more detailed choices will be presented. If the user indicated that they did not like a particular category, no list of specific items will be presented.

Level of deprivation of most preferred items. Once a user has chosen his or her most preferred items, the user is then asked how much more he or she would like to receive that item. For example, if the user chose ice cream as a favorite snack or dessert, he or she would be asked "How much more would you like to eat ice cream?"

Response format. The response format requires that an individual make a choice for each question. The specific wording of the response choice will depend on which question is given and is either a list of specific items or a single response scale. The response scale wording was influenced by the responses obtained in the pilot study. General category questions that typically had strong, clear preferences have a "Yes" or "No" response choice; items that were not as clearly distinguished have a "Very much," "A little," or "Not at all" response scale. For example, strong preferences were found when participants were asked "What sport do you like to play?" Approximately 20% of the participants responded "none."

A menu list is given for the specific item questions. For the questions regarding satiation or deprivation, the users are given the choice of wanting something "A lot more," "A little more," or "I _____ (ex., eat) it enough already."

General lists. Following all the questions about various reinforcers, the items selected as most preferred will be presented by reinforcer category. Also, the items in which the individual indicated that they liked, and that they would like to have a lot more of, is presented in a list (across reinforcer categories). The user then chooses from these lists his or her overall most preferred items.

Report. A report is generated that presents all items that the user had chosen as most preferred, and those items that he or she had indicated as wanting to receive more often. These items are organized by the response given (ex., likes very much, wants a lot more, has enough already), and by the type of reinforcer category (ex., by things to eat, social activities, etc.). The report also shows the overall most preferred reinforcers for that individual, answers to specific questions, items added to the assessment, indication of a preference for a delay in reinforcement, etc. The total number of items selected is also presented, as this may be relevant as information regarding feelings of depression, hopelessness, etc.

General Discussion

The MARA program has not been formally tested. However, most of the individuals who have completed MARA have indicated that it was enjoyable to take. Normally intelligent children that read well were able to use it independently (once it was on the screen) at age 9. It has been successfully given to a 4-year-old with slight rewording of the questions, with the examiner entering the responses. Thus, realistically, this program can most likely be used with assistance of the examiner at a 5 or 6 year old level, and independently (depending on reading and computer abilities) at a 10-year old level.

One of the intentions in the development of MARA was to be able to use the results of the assessment in a way that is useful for the individual. However, the true test of what is and is not a reinforcer lies in its application. What is reinforcing at one time, may not be reinforcing at another. For these reasons, it may be best to use the MARA just prior to selecting a reinforcer. In addition, individuals could review their printout and indicate what they think would be the most effective reinforcers. The MARA provides the user with an individualized selection of reinforcers at any given time, for any given purpose.

Much more testing is needed before definitive conclusions can be made regarding MARA. However, as it stands, MARA can provide a teacher, mental health professional, technician, etc., with a thorough list of their client's stated preferences, which can then be used in changing the client's behavior, activity selection, assessing treatment goals, etc.

Software Availability

A copy of the software can be obtained by writing: Dr. Vatterott, (MARA), Missouri Institute of Mental Health, 5247 Fyler, St Louis, MO 63139. The software is also on the Testing Station BBS (See Chapter 2). The questionnaire driver used (Knowledge Pro) is available commercially through Knowledge Garden, Inc., 473A Malden Bridge Dr., Nassau, NY 12123. (518) 776-3000.

REFERENCES

Atkinson, R. P., Jenson, W. R., Rovner, L., Cameron, S., Van Wagenen, L., & Petersen, B. P. (1984). Brief report: Validation of the Autism Reinforcer Checklist for children. Journal of Autism and Developmental Disorders, 14, 429-433.

Bihm, E. M. (1989). Reinforcer responsiveness check list. (Available from Elson M. Bihm, Department of Psychology and Counseling, University of Central Arkansas, 72032).

Cautela, J. R., & Brion-Meisels, L. (1979). A Children's Reinforcement Survey Schedule. Psychological Reports, 44, 327-338.

Cautela, J. R., & Kastenbaum, R. (1967). A Reinforcement Survey Schedule for use in therapy, training, and research. Psychological Reports, 20, 1115-1130.

Cartwright, C. A., & Cartwright, G. P. (1970). Determining the motivational systems of individual children. Teaching Exceptional Children, 2, 143-149.

Dewhurst, D. L. T., & Cautela, J. R. (1980). A proposed reinforcement survey schedule for special needs children. Journal of Behavior Therapy and Experimental Psychiatry, 11, 109-112.

Durand, V. M., & Crimmins, D. B. (1988). Identifying the variables maintaining self-injurious behavior. Journal of Autism and Developmental Disorders, 18, 99-117.

Hall, R. V., & Hall, M. C. (1980). How to select reinforcers. Lawrence, KS: H & H Enterprises.

Heron, T. E. (1987). Operant reinforcement. In J. O. Cooper, T. E. Heron, & W. L. Heward (Eds.), Applied behavior analysis (pp. 254-274). Columbus, OH: Merrill.

Keat, D. B. (1974). Survey schedule of rewards for children. Psychological Reports, 35, 287-293.

Phillips, D., Fischer, S. C., & Singh, R. (1977). A Children's Reinforcement Survey Schedule. Journal of Behavior Therapy and Experimental Psychiatry, 8, 131-134.

Timberlake, W., & Allison, J. (1974). Response deprivation: An empirical approach to instrumental performance. Psychological Review, 81, 146-164.

Willis, T. J., & LaVigna, G. (1987). Reinforcement inventory. In T. J. Willis, G. W. LaVigna, & A. M. Donnellan (Eds.), Behavior Assessment Guide (pp. 1-6). Los Angeles: Institute for Applied Behavioral Analysis.

An Automated Screening Schedule for Mental Health Centers

Kimberly A. Sloan
Keith Eldridge
Richard Evenson

KEYWORDS. Computerized patient testing, mental health software, community mental health

BACKGROUND

As the mental health field increasingly relies on computers to manage administrative information, computers are becoming a familiar aspect of the work setting (Parley & Cohen, 1984). Yet clinical applications of computer technology have been much slower to be accepted (Gorodezky & Hedlund, 1982). Many view computerized assessment as an under-utilized resource that can provide immediate, inexpensive information to clinicians about psychological symptoms and personality dynamics (Ben-Porath & Butcher, 1986).

Several studies have found that clients report favorable attitudes toward automated testing and often prefer it to manual test administration (Angle, Ellinwood, Hay, Hohsen, & Hay, 1977; Barnett, 1982; Erdman, Greist, Klien, Jefferson, & Getto, 1981; Skinner & Allen, 1983). The use of automated assessment as part of a standard clinical intake process is therefore not likely to impede and may enhance the therapeutic process. Research suggests that clients of-

Kimberly A. Sloan, PhD, completed the program while a Post Doctoral Fellow at Missouri Institute of Mental Health at 5247 Flyer, St. Louis, MO 63139. Keith Eldridge, PhD, programmed the schedule. Richard Evenson, PhD, is a faculty member at the Institute.

ten feel more comfortable reporting sensitive personal information to a computer than to a clinician during an intake interview (Lucas, Card, Knill-Jones, Watkinson, & Cream, 1976; Lucas, Mullins, Luna, & McInroy, 1977; Skinner & Allen, 1983; Slack & Slack, 1977).

Many studies have examined comparability between paper and pencil and automated test administration. Generally high test-retest reliability and no significant mean score differences between manual and computer administration were found (Bartran & Bayliss, 1984; Ben-Porath & Butcher, 1986; Davis & Cowles, 1989; Elwood, 1969, Katz & Dalby, 1981; McLeod, Griffiths, Bigelow, & Yingling, 1982). Standardized clinical measures can therefore be automated with the expectation that the same validity and reliability information can be demonstrated on the computer.

PROGRAM DEVELOPMENT

This program was designed to meet the needs of a community mental health center. Meetings were held with administrators and clinicians from the Four County Mental Health Center in St. Charles, Missouri to define the goals of the automated screening schedule.

The center is moving toward providing briefer treatment to reduce the amount of time clients spend on the waiting list before receiving services. Most clients are women, many of whom have suffered various kinds of childhood abuse that is often not discovered until a solid therapeutic relationship is established. In addition, many clients have particular problems with self-esteem and intimacy.

DESCRIPTION OF THE PROGRAM

The automated screening schedule was programmed in Clipper 87. The main menu allows for activation of the full battery or access to the particular tests. Options allow for printing the report and access to the database. Prior to accessing the database files, however, a security code must be entered.

Questions are presented in a multiple choice format except for the demographic questions. These require some typing. A "help" screen was developed to aid clients should they have difficulty remembering the instructions. All clients complete the same battery of questions until a branching segment asks whether victimization has occurred. If acknowledged, further questions are asked about it, otherwise the program skips to the consumer satisfaction questions.

DESCRIPTION OF THE SCREENING SCHEDULE

The goal of the screening schedule was to provide client information to clinicians prior to the first session. The information generally focuses on symptoms, self-esteem, and relationships. After collecting basic demographic information, the screening schedule asks clients to choose all that apply from sixteen reasons for coming to the clinic. None of the above is presented as an option.

The automated schedule includes three well established self-rating scales that employ a Likert-Scale format. The Heming and Courtney (1984) self-esteem scale measures five aspects of self-esteem in thirty-six questions. The factors are self-regard, social confidence, physical appearance, physical abilities, and school abilities. The six questions comprising the school factor were dropped. A five item social desirability scale (Hays, Hayashi, & Stewart, 1989) was incorporated into the self-esteem measure (see Appendix A & B). The intimate bonds scale (Wilhelm & Parker, 1988) has twenty-four items that measure perceived care and control in one's most significant relationship. The St. Louis Symptom Checklist is an empirically derived ninety question scale that assesses felt distress on eleven subscales. It was developed from the Missouri Institute of Psychiatry's computerized state hospital database.

An automated interview segment asks about physical and sexual victimization. If the client acknowledges physical or sexual abuse, questions are asked to indicate: when the abuse occurred; the age of the abuser; who the abuser was; and whether the abuse was reported to anyone.

The impact of life events scale (Horowitz, Wilner, & Alvarez, 1985) is administered to assess the clients style of coping with trauma. This fifteen item questionnaire has two factors or styles of coping with trauma. The intrusion subscale includes items like repetitive thoughts, memories, and nightmares about the trauma. The avoidance factor measures the tendency to put it "out of one's mind" or avoid reminders associated with it.

At the end of the automated battery, clients are asked questions regarding consumer comfort and satisfaction. This nine item scale was adapted from the well known CS-8, the most widely used consumer satisfaction scale.

AUTOMATED SCREENING SCHEDULE REPORT

All scores referred to in the report are shown on a scale of 1-100, with a mean of 50 and a standard deviation of 10. This is a T scale. Like the MMPI, a score of 70 is viewed as significant. That is, a client's score is compared to the group mean presented in the literature for that test. A score of 70 would indicate that the client scored two standard deviations above the published group mean for the test.

The social desirability scale questions are used to make a statement at the beginning of the report about the client's level of defensiveness. A score above the mean places the client in the defensive or not open and frank category of test taking attitudes.

The report also lists descriptive information about the client. Presenting problems are listed after the defensiveness section. For the St. Louis symptom checklist, items that were endorsed as being moderately bothersome during the past week are listed for the eleven subscales. There is also a section that lists the critical items that were endorsed with respect to injury of self or others. The descriptive information was presented to alert clinicians to specific client complaints. In order to provide specific information about intimate relationship concerns, items that were endorsed in the most negative direction on the Intimate Bonds scale are also listed.

The automated screening report provides both quantitative and descriptive information about clients. All information gathered from the battery is presented in the report except the information from the consumer satisfaction questions.

TESTING OF THE AUTOMATED
SCREENING SCHEDULE

Sixty-one clients were administered the automated screening schedule before their first clinical interview at the Four County Mental Health Agency. It took clients twenty to thirty minutes to complete the battery. Only one client did not finish the battery, complaining that he could not concentrate. Several clients who completed the testing were in the mild range of mental retardation. No clients complained about the testing and only a few declined to participate. Formal analysis of the consumer satisfaction data has not been completed.

A secretary was trained to administer the battery to clients. The secretary reported that she did not have any difficulty administering the tests and did not feel that it inconvenienced her routine.

Informal feedback from the clinicians indicated that they found the information quite helpful. Several clinicians indicated that the information allowed them to explore sensitive areas with clients earlier than had been their customary practice.

A formal statistical analysis of the data collected on the sixty-one clients is in the process of being completed. This information should provide quantative evidence to support the informal feedback from clients that they felt the testing was easy to complete and helpful to their treatment.

CONCLUSIONS

The Automated Screening Schedule was found to run smoothly and usefully within the community mental health agency where it was tested. It provides quick informative summaries of client symptoms and feelings about self and closest other. In addition, it provides information about physical and sexual abuse. This issue has received increasing prominence in the mental health field but little sound research has been published. The ability to compile a computerized database that this program offers allows for systematic investigation of this issue as well as many others.

NEXT STEPS

Once the data from the initial sample is analyzed, the sample norms will be compared with published norms. published norms for the scales were used to derive the standard scores that are printed in the automated screening schedule report. If significant differences in the norms emerge, adjustments will need to be made in the program.

Before modifications in the program are made, however, it would be useful to gather data from other populations where the program is being used. At this point, we are inviting outpatient mental health centers to try the program. We would be happy to provide a copy of the program, hoping that center will provide us with a copy of their database. A copy of the program may be obtained by writing to the first author.

REFERENCES

Briere, J. (1988). Symptomatology associated with childhood sexual victimization in a nonclinical adult sample. Child Abuse & Neglect, 12, 51-59.

Butcher, J. N., Keller, L. S., & Bacon, S. F. (1985). Current developments and future directions in computerized personality assessment. Journal of Consulting and Clinical Psychology, 53(6), 803-815.

Crowne, D. P., & Marlowe, D. (1960). A new scale of social desirability independent of psychopathology. Journal of Consulting Psychology, 24, 349-354.

Davis, C., & Cowles, M. (1989). Automated psychological testing: Method of administration, need for approval, and measures of anxiety. Educational and Psychological Measurement, 49, 311-320.

Elwood, D. L. (1969). Automation of psychological testing. American Psychologist, 24, 287-288.

Finkelhor, D., & Browne, A. (1985). The traumatic impact of child sexual abuse: A conceptualization. American Journal of Orthopsychiatry, 55(4), 530-541.

Fleming, J. S., & Courtney, B. E. (1984). The dimensionality of self esteem: II. Hierarchical facet model for revised measurement scales. Journal of Personality and Social Psychology, 46(2), 404-421.

Fromuth, M. E., & Burkhart, B. R. (1989). Long-term psychological correlates of childhood sexual abuse in two samples of college men. Child Abuse & Neglect, 13, 533-542.

Hays, R. D., Hayashi, T., & Stewart, A. T. (1989). A five item measure of socially desirable response set. Educational and Psychological Measurement, 49, 629-636.

Hedlund, J. L., & Vieweg, B. W. (1988). Automation in psychological testing. Psychiatric Annals, 18(4), 217-227.

Hedlund, J. L., Vieweg, B. W., & Cho, D. W. (1985). Mental health computing in the 1980's: I. General information systems and clinical documentation. Computers in Human Services, 1(1), 3-33.

Hedlund, J. L., Vieweg, B. W., & Cho, D. W. (1985). Mental health computing in the 1980's: II. Clinical Applications. Computers in Human Services, 1(2), 1-29.

Horowitz, M. J., Wilner, N., & Alvarez, W. (1979). Impact of event scales: A measure of subjective stress. Psychosomatic Medicine, 41, 209-218.

Jacobson, A., & Richardson, B. (1987). Assault experiences of 100 psychiatric inpatients: Evidence of the need for routine inquiry. American Journal of Psychiatry, 144, 908-913.

Katz, L., & Dalby, J. T. (1981). Computer and manual administration of the Eysenck personality inventory. Journal of Clinical Psychology, 37(3), 586-588.

Lister, E. D. (1982). Forced Silence: A neglected dimension of trauma. American Journal of Psychiatry, 139(7), 872-875.

Lucas, R. W., Mullin, P. J., Luna, C. B. X., & McInroy, D. C. (1977). Psychiatrists and a computer as interrogators of patients with alcohol related illnesses: A comparison. British Journal of Psychiatry, 131, 160-167.

McLeod, D. R., Griffiths, R. R., Bigelow, G. E., & Yingling, J. (1982). Computer Technology: An automated version of the digit symbol substitution test (DSST). Behavior Research Methods & Instrumentation, 14(5), 463-466.

Newsted, P. R. (1985). Paper versus online presentations of subjective questionnaires. International Journal of Man-Machine Studies, 23, 231-247.

Skinner, H. A., & Allen, B. A. (1983). Does the computer make a difference? Computerized versus face-to-face self report assessment of alcohol, drug, and tobacco use. Journal of Consulting and Clinical Psychology, 51(2), 267-275.

Thompson, J. A., & Wilson, S. L. (1982). Automated psychological testing. International Journal of Man-Machine Studies, 17(3), 279-289.

Van Leeuwenn, K. (1988). Resistances in the treatment of a sexually molested 6-year-old girl. Institute of Psycho-Analysis, 15, 149-156.

Wilhelm, K., & Parker, G. (1988). The development of measure of intimate bonds. Psychological Medicine, 18, 225-234.

Zilberg, N. J., Weiss, D. S., & Horowitz, M. J. (1982). Impact of event scale: A cross validation study and some empirical evidence supporting a conceptual model of stress response syndromes. Journal of Consulting and Clinical Psychology, 50(3), 407-414.

Psychiatric Paperwork Enhancement Through Quasi Automated Office Systems Development

Carol A. Zawacky
Vladimir G. Levit
Muzaffar M. Khan
Anjan Bhattacharyya

KEYWORDS. Computerized medical records, computer assisted treatment planning, word processing, mental health software

OVERVIEW

State of the art computer technology is able to assist overburdened clinicians (Taintor, 1987) in minimizing duplicate paperwork tasks by using word processing systems. Several treatment centers have made successful attempts to automate the psychiatric record, focusing on both clinical assessment documents (Gifford & Maberry, 1979; Mezzich, Dow, Ganguli, Munetz, Zettler-Segal, 1986; Hammond & Munnecke, 1984; Chang, 1987) and comprehensive treatment plans (Gifford & Maberry, 1979; Mezzich et al., 1986; Hammond & Munnecke, 1984). These automation systems used complex data base management software packages which required extensive computer programming and were very expensive to fund. Ormiston, Barrett, Binder, and Molyneuz (1989), however, devel-

Carol A. Zawacky, PhD, is a psychologist at the Rockland Psychiatric Center, Orangeburg, NY 10962. Anjan Bhattacharyya, MS, is Director of the Microcomputing Department, Quality Assurance Division, at Rockland Psychiatric Center, Orangeburg, NY 10962.

63

oped a partially computerized treatment planning program using a word processing software package in a personal computer.

This article describes an automation system which the authors piloted in an extended care services unit at a state inpatient psychiatric facility. The computerization system began in 1988 with one treatment team using word processing software in a microcomputer to write psychiatric and psychological assessments, monthly patient progress notes, and comprehensive treatment plan reviews. Once proven to be effective in reducing time spent in these tasks, the authors sought to systematically streamline and enhance a number of psychiatric documents.

COMPUTERIZED ASSESSMENTS AND CORE HISTORY

The word processing system which was developed incorporated three main goals — (1) to attempt to eliminate the duplication of information in initial and annual Psychiatric and Social assessments, particularly in regard to the historical data, (2) to improve the quality and consistency of initial and annual Psychiatric and Social assessments by incorporating a detailed legend, and (3) to semi-automate the psychiatric paperwork documentation in such a way as to minimize the duplicate information processing needed when writing a variety of psychiatric summaries or documents.

To these ends, structured Psychiatric and Social assessment forms were revised to enhance automation. These assessments were edited by the Chiefs of Psychiatry and Social Work, respectively, as a major and very useful revision of current O.M.H. forms. They were consequently approved by the Medical Staff Organization (M.S.O.) Medical Records Committee and Executive Committee for a period of trial, in consultation with the Clinical Director.

The first step of the restructuring process led to two versions of the Psychiatric and Social Assessments, namely, an initial assessment and an annual update. It was felt that the focus is a bit different when a Psychiatric or Social assessment is done in an inpatient or outpatient unit for a first admission as opposed to subsequent annual updates. The annual updates include the treatment course since the last assessment. Several new items were added to the Psychiatric Assessments to capture issues like psychopharmacological interventions in chronological order.

The next step incorporated a very detailed legend (Kaplan & Sadock, 1985) into both initial and annual versions of the Psychiatric and Social Assessments (see Appendix A) to enhance the clarity and comprehensiveness of the documents. Most clinical assessment items typically ask the writer for information in a narrative style, which leaves it up to the writer to decide what information needs to be included in each item. There is a great deal of variation among writers in the information they provide, depending on level of sophistication with the assessment process, training, degree of disciplined thinking, and perhaps memory as well. In our experience in piloting this legend in the annual Psychiatric assessment, the structure provided by the legend has improved the quality of the document. In terms of the automation system, this legend can be incorporated in the file as a "document comment" which does not appear on the printed copy which goes into the medical record.

In terms of our second goal, we initially attempted to develop a system of merge and macro functions to transfer historical data from one assessment to another: i.e., from the initial Social Assessment to the initial Psychiatric Assessment; from the initial Psychiatric Assessment to the annual Psychiatric Assessment; from the initial Social Assessment to the annual Social Assessment. However, we found that the level of computer programming expertise and staff time needed to develop this system was quite extensive. This stumbling block eventually led us to look in other directions. We appreciated certain strengths in the recent draft of the Office of Mental Health Outpatient Record Prototype (Forquer, 1991). Following this lead, a "Core History" document (see Appendix B) was separated out of the assessments. This Core History document contains historical data for a patient which is gathered on first admission and then updated annually or as new information becomes available. We found this to be an effective tool to further reduce the redundancy of the duplicate information processing found in the Social and Psychiatric assessments.

If the clinician wishes to have any additional information transferred from an initial assessment to an annual assessment, or from the previous annual assessment to a current assessment, a word processing "move" function can be carried out. The Core History and Psychiatric/Social Assessment documents can be typed directly on the computer either by the psychiatrist or social worker or by secretarial staff who type from a tape or handwritten assessment. A first draft of the document can be printed for any necessary editing and for review with the clinical supervisor.

AUTOMATION OF OTHER PSYCHIATRIC DOCUMENTS

Many psychiatric documents are prepared during a patient's hospitalization, such as the Discharge Summary, Application for Court Retention, Application for Court Authorization to Medicate Over Patient Objection, Presentations for Supervisory Case Reviews, and Authorization to use approved drugs for unlabeled purposes, etc. In terms of our third goal, we feel that these reports can be expedited by the transfer of information from the Psychiatric Assessment or Core History using a word processing move function. The O.M.H. Discharge Summary form was revised (see Appendix C) to facilitate the transfer of relevant information (items 1 through 7) taken from the computerized Core History and Psychiatric Assessment forms. The computerized Discharge Summary form contains word processing "document comments" placed under each of the first seven items. These comments give the typist instructions on how to move items from the computerized Core History and Psychiatric Assessment and where to place them in the Discharge Summary. These comments do not appear in the printed document. A detailed legend was also added to the remaining sections of the Discharge Summary, which are then completed by the psychiatrist (the treatment course and final discharge diagnosis) and the social worker (aftercare plans). Similarly, other psychiatric documents which are routinely prepared could be restructured to facilitate automation. Since the clinician is no longer spending time in gathering duplicate information, this time can be translated into improving quality of clinical documentation.

AUTOMATION OF ASSESSMENT RECOMMENDATIONS

In an effort to explore the utility of using word processing software to facilitate the often tedious process of treatment planning
conceptualization and writing, Drs. Levit and Zawacky developed a
first draft of a text of psychiatric syndromes along with suggestions
for goals and methods. Each psychiatric syndrome and its accompanying goals/treatment methods was stored as a word processing
"macro." The psychiatrist would thereby invoke the macro which
pertained to the patient's clinical syndrome into the Psychiatric assessment under the Treatment Recommendations section. The problems and goals would be individualized/edited according to the patient's specific clinical condition, often resulting in several short
term objectives. Further review and individualization would be
done at the multidisciplinary treatment planning meeting and the
final product would be incorporated into the Comprehensive Treatment Plan. A number of the more frequently diagnosed medical
conditions were also included, e.g., hypertension, diabetes, obe-
sity, etc.

In developing this system, it is important to note that a good deal
of clinical thinking was necessary to address the main weaknesses
of several pre-existing treatment planning manuals. We wondered
why these systems of objectives and methods were not used by
clinical staff (who desperately searched for help with treatment plan
writing), even though they appeared to be quite elaborate. In our
analysis, the main weakness of these manuals was that they listed
isolated symptoms with accompanying methods for treating them.
These systems failed to incorporate the clinical conceptualization of
symptoms as part of a main psychopathological syndrome. In psychiatric practice we treat the syndrome, not the symptom, although
we are able to look at changes in particular signs or symptoms as
windows to determine whether there is clinical improvement or deterioration in the syndromal pathology. We found that this clinical
approach to treatment planning greatly facilitated understanding of
the patient among the multidisciplinary treatment team and made
the task of treatment plan writing a great deal easier and enhanced
the quality of the treatment plan.

FUTURE DEVELOPMENTS

Clinicians as Psychiatric Application Developers

In the past three years, we have gained experience in developing and using a variety of computer software applications in our service. In addition to the previously described word processing systems, we have also developed a database management system, which was piloted in one unit. We found that recently available database management packages allowed us (clinicians) to create and use a sophisticated database in a brief time without having computer programming experience.

It is essential, in any agency, that any software developed should have the full support of clinical and administrative staff. We have found that it is necessary to involve the clinical staff in the development of these applications to engender a sense of ownership that comes from being involved from the inception of a project. Craig et al. (1982) found that, in spite of a high quality software product, a significant number of the clinical staff of a mental health facility were quite resistive to implementing a treatment planning system since they perceived it as being imposed upon them, rather than having a perception of ownership. An additional liability was that senior staff were unfamiliar with the benefits of the system and there was no clear administrative mandate for its implementation.

In order to generate a sense of excitement and ownership among the clinical and senior administrative leaders at the facility, we have established a Clinical Computer Applications Management Committee of the M.S.O., which has indeed generated significant interest in the psychiatric staff. Under the auspices of the former facility Acting Clinical Director (M.K.), a Medical Staff Organization was established a few years ago which enabled medical/clinical staff to not only voice their professional opinion as to what is clinically sound but to put clinicians in decision and policy making positions. It is our hope that this committee will further develop and effectively implement clinically relevant and high quality word processing and database applications which lead to a substantial enhancement in the quality of treatment services at our facility.

Currently, we are in the process of piloting the word processing system in several services. In our experience it is essential to take small steps in piloting an application, rather than effecting the entire facility at one time. We chose units with a young, chronically mentally ill patient population. Therein, the patient movement was much more stable as opposed to an acute admissions service. This also gave us access to broader numbers and types of problems which would not be found in a geriatric service. We identified one clinical treatment team to pilot the application, and after they developed proficiency in it, we then encouraged other teams to join in. The outcome has been very dramatic. We will be conducting trial runs in one selected team in other units, including admissions, geriatrics, and outpatient services, as identified by their Chief Medical Officers. Our hope is that if this system is eventually implemented throughout the facility, at the time that a patient moves between various inpatient units or from inpatient to outpatient services, relevant word processing and database information will be transferred on a diskette to the receiving service. This would translate into improved continuity of care since clinical assessment and Core History documents would be legible and need only to be updated with any new pertinent information.

Treatment Plans

Clinical assessments lead to the development of treatment plans, which must be specific in terms of patient outcome and treatment methodology. Automation can help to ensure such specificity by having guidelines or menus in the software (Taintor, 1987). In order to develop clinically pertinent treatment plans within the context of a multidisciplinary team structure, which are in compliance with JCAHO, HCFA, and other regulatory agencies, several skills are required. Excellent clinical skills as well as highly organized and critical thinking are necessary to develop a case formulation in the context of historical and presenting data.

Finding a combination of the clinical skills, command of English, critical thinking, and organizational skills which are necessary to produce a clinically sound treatment plan in one person or in a clinical team is rare. In a large organization such as ours with ever-shrinking resources, it is indeed an arduous task to train our clinical staff in all of these skills.

In addition to the ability to conceptualize the clinical problems as manifested by the patient in holistic, historic, and current context, and to identify broad major clinical syndromes, the clinician has to focus his thinking in a problem-oriented way. The clinician has to identify the specific problem or problems which are keeping this patient at the current level of care. We work under severe pressure of fiscal and regulatory agencies, which demand that we discharge/ transfer patients, as soon as possible, to less restrictive, less labor intensive, and less costly settings. This task requires us to identify problems, to prioritize them in the context of discharge planning, and then to develop goal/objectives and interventions which are measurable. We in the mental health field, however, tend to think in a global manner. Other disciplines of medicine are much more specific and goal oriented.

The work done to date in piloting computerized psychiatric assessment treatment recommendations in one treatment team has been an initial attempt to deal with the elusive process of treatment planning. To further develop our thinking on the utility of automating treatment plans, we reviewed those plans developed in our facility during the last six months which were found to be in compliance by our QA department. It became evident that the number of main clinical syndromes is rather small, perhaps about two dozen. Therefore, if we attempt to conceptualize a computer program which would incorporate the main clinical syndromes encountered in our facility, it could very likely be manageable. Each clinical syndrome could have about four goals, each goal could have about four objectives, and each objective could have as many methods as members in the treatment team.

For example, this program would incorporate the following lists:

1. Syndrome list
2. Goal list as sub-menu of each syndrome
3. Objective list as sub-menu of each goal
4. Method list as sub-menu of each objective

Let us suppose we are dealing with the paranoid syndrome and the core problem is refusal of all treatment interventions. We can translate this core problem into a menu of goals. One of them could be chosen and modified as necessary. The wording and outline of this goal will guide the clinician's thinking.

Note that in order to develop a computerized treatment planning system, a systematic analysis must be done of all the steps involved in the treatment planning process, from its inception to completion. The development of such a system necessitates a great deal of clinical thinking and computerization work, as well as the patience to refine, debug, and pilot the system, which leads to further refinement, debugging, and piloting. These efforts may be quite worthwhile, however, in view of the fact that the treatment plan is the main focus of accrediting agency reviews, and in a sense, our clinical work is perceived as succeeding or failing according to the outcome of these surveys.

In the era of ever-shrinking resources at all levels, and concurrent reduction in the work force, it is crucial that we minimize the time spent in paperwork tasks. It is our hope that the resulting time efficiency of professional staff, as well as the improved quality of clinical assessments for treatment planning, will lead to enhanced quality and consistency of clinical interventions and successful treatment outcomes for our patients.

CONCLUSIONS

Since the clinical practice of psychology or psychiatry requires a great deal of writing (i.e., assessments, mental status reports, case histories, consultation reports, progress notes) much of this work can and should be done on the word processor (Lieff, 1987). We have attempted to use computer technology to reduce the amount of time clinicians spend in paperwork tasks, as well as to enhance the quality of these documents. We feel that the word processing system which was developed for use in our facility proved to be quite useful in the pilot settings. We have yet to accomplish the larger task of implementing the system facility-wide and evaluating it systematically over time.

A major advantage of this psychiatric paperwork reduction system in its generalizability to other mental health settings. The core documents are comprised of relatively standardized items, which are not facility specific. Therefore a new user could directly implement this system with only minor modification as desired.

Our system of automating assessment recommendations for treatment planning appeared to support the concept of the syndromal approach as the basis for developing a clinically sound treatment plan. We used a popular, off-the-shelf word processor with good results. Further advancements might consider the use of more sophisticated word processors that allow interacting with a database or perhaps using a database front end with a series of menus and submenus.

REFERENCES

American Psychiatric Association. (1987). *Diagnostic and Statistical Manual of Mental Disorders, Third Edition-Revised*. Washington, DC: American Psychiatric Association.

Chang, M. (1987). Clinician-Entered Computerized Psychiatric Triage Records. *Hospital and Community Psychiatry, 38*(6), 652-656.

Craig, T., Volaski, V., DiStefano, O., Alexander, M., Kadyzewski, P., Crawford, J., & Richardson, M. (1982). Automating the treatment planning process: How? Why? For whom? In: Blum, B. (Ed.) *Proceedings of the Sixth Annual Symposium on Computer Applications in Medical Care*. New York: Institute of Electrical and Electronics Engineers.

Forquer, S.L. (1991). *UCR Redesign Project Outpatient Record Prototype: Forms, Highlights, And Instructions*. Office of Mental Health.

Gifford, S. & Maberry, D. (1979). An Integrated System for Computerized Patient Records. *Hospital and Community Psychiatry, 30*(8), 532-535.

Hammond, K. & Munnecke, T. (1984). A Computerized Psychiatric Treatment Planning System. *Hospital and Community Psychiatry, 35*(2), 160-163.

Kaplan, H., & Sadock, B. (1985). *Modern Synopsis of Comprehensive Textbook of Psychiatry/IV*. Baltimore, MD: Williams & Wilkins.

Lieff, J. (1987). *Computer Applications in Psychiatry*. Washington D.C., American Psychiatric Press.

Mezzich, J., Dow, J., Ganguli, R., Munetz, M., & Zettler-Segal, M. (1986). Computerized Initial and Discharge Evaluations. In J. Mezzich (Ed.), *Clinical Care and Information Systems in Psychiatry* (pp. 13-58). Washington, DC: American Psychiatric Press, Inc.

Ormiston, S., Barrett, N., Binder, R., & Molyneux, V. (1989). A Partially Computerized Treatment Plan. *Hospital and Community Psychiatry*, *40*(5), 531-533.

Taintor, Z. (1987). Chronic Mental Illness and Computer Uses. In Greist, J., Carroll, J., Erdman, H., Klein, M., & Wurster, C. (Eds.), *Research in mental health computer applications: Directions for the future* (pp. 89-92). Washington, D.C.: Superintendent of Documents, U.S. Government Printing Office.

WordPerfect, Version 5.1. (1989). Orem, Utah, WordPerfect Corporation.

APPENDIX A

PSYCH.INI Rev. 6/9/91

Rockland Psychiatric Center

PSYCHIATRIC ASSESSMENT (INITIAL)

INSTRUCTIONS:
  — Review and co-sign the core history.
  — Complete by the due date of first treatment plan meeting.
  — Update continuously during the course of treatment. Use continuation sheets

Patient Data: Lastname, Firstname, MI
  C#, DOB
  Unit/Ward, Sex

I. CURRENT MENTAL STATUS EXAMINATION

1. *GENERAL APPEARANCE*: (Sex, race, personal hygiene and grooming status; estimate of age in context of the stated age, level of psychomotor activity; any abnormal movements and gait; mannerisms, tics, gestures and any other peculiar behavior)

2. *ATTITUDE/BEHAVIOR RAPPORT:* (Patient's level of cooperation, capacity to relate to the examiner and ability to engage and develop rapport. Whether patient is comfortable, ill at ease, pleasant, friendly, cooperative, defensive, guarded, hostile, able to stay for the time scheduled, restless, demanding, pacing and estimate of his/her ability to develop rapport with the examiner and level of engagement in the process)

3. *THOUGHT PROCESS:* (Stream of thought; Productivity; Overabundance of ideas, Paucity of ideas; Flight of ideas; Rapid, pressured, and hesitant thinking; Spontaneity; Continuity of thought, coherent, incoherent; Relevant, irrelevant to the topics discussed; Thought blocking; Loose associations; Clang associations; Circumstantiality; Tangentiality; Clarity of speech; Goal directedness; Rambling; Evasive; Perseverative; Distractibility; Word salad; Neologisms; etc.)

4. *THOUGHT CONTENTS:*

A. *Preoccupation:* (Include predominant concerns patient is occupied with, e.g., about illness, environmental problems, family and other social and interpersonal problems, discharge, transfer, pass card and other privileges)

B. *Delusional Ideation:* (*Include nature and contents of delusional ideas*) fixed, systematized, organized, disorganized, loose, persecutory, grandiose, nihilistic, somatic, delusions of control, ideas of reference or influence, thought control, thought insertion, thought withdrawal, thought broadcasting, patently bizarre, mood congruent/incongruent, *degree of patient's conviction as to its validity, and its effect on his life and behavior*. Give examples in patient's own words in parenthesis)

C. *Obsessions, Compulsions:* (Include contents of obsessive thoughts and intensity of affect; contents of compulsive acts and affective intensity, and degree of control on patient's behavior)

D. *Perceptual Disturbances:* (*Include illusions and various types of hallucinations;* visual, auditory, tactile, gustatory, olfactory, command hallucinations, etc., *it's contents*; derogatory, persecutory, grandiose, command hallucinations, etc., *its frequency, intensity, duration, and circumstances of the occurrence. Patient's conviction as to its validity*; Egosyntonic; Egodystonic; Its influence on pt.'s life and behavior; Experiences of depersonalization, derealization, excessive feeling of detachment from oneself or the environment. Give examples in pt.'s words in parenthesis)

E. *Suicidal, Homicidal Ideas and Behavior:* (Include the theme; Intensity of the impulse; Precipitating factors; Degree of Control; History of such behavior in the past; Homicidal ideation directed to person(s), objects, intended victims and pt.'s reasons. Use pt.'s own words as much as possible)

F. *Impulse Control:* (Include pt.'s ability to control aggressive, hostile, sexual impulses under ordinary living conditions (at home and/or on the ward, etc.)

5. *MOOD, FEELINGS, and AFFECT:*

A. *Mood:* (A pervasive and sustained emotion that colors the person's perception of the world over days and weeks. Include depth, intensity, duration, fluctuation of mood. Give detailed account of associated clinical features if the pt. has a mood disorder)

B. *Affect:* (Outward manifestation of emotion associated with expressed ideas. Restricted, depressed, blunted, shallow, constricted, labile, range of the affect. Its appropriateness, congruity and incongruity, to the thought content, the culture, and setting)

C. *Anxiety, Panic, Phobias, Somatization, Hypochondriasis and Dissociative symptoms:* (Include phobias, concern and anxiety related to it; Generalized anxiety symptoms and panic attacks; precipitating circumstances, defensive systems or life style patient has developed to minimize panic attacks; Somatization tendencies; Hypochondriacal symptoms, give specific examples; Dissociative symptoms such as depersonalization, derealization, conversion disorder and multiple personality disorder; Antisocial urges; etc.)

6. *COGNITIVE FUNCTIONS EXAMINATION:*

A. *Sensorium and Level of Consciousness:* (Include clarity of sensorium, alertness, cloudiness, lability and variability)

B. *Orientation:* (Include orientation to place, person, and time. Give examples)

C. *Memory Functions:*
C1. *Registration, Retention, and Immediate Recall:* (Ability to repeat 6 numbers after auditory or visual exposure, first forward and then backwards; Registration, retention, and recall of three objects immediately, after one and five minutes)

C2. *Attention and Calculation:* (Ability for focused behavior; Distractibility; Ability to calculate simple problems; Subtracting Serial Sevens, Serial Fives, Serial Threes, etc.)

C3. *Recent/Short-term Memory:* (Memory of the past few days, what did patient do today, yesterday and the day before)

C4. *Remote/Long-term/Past Memory:* (Include date of birth, place of birth, important events occurring when patient was young, names of schools attended, etc. Give examples. Evaluate both early life memories and intermediate life memories)

C5. *Recognition Memory:* (Include ability to recognize family members and caregivers)
D. *Language Comprehension, Expression and Execution of Command:* (Include command of language and comprehension. Ask patient to name certain objects such as pencil and watch; Have the patient repeat "no ifs, ands, or buts;" Follow a three-step command (i.e., take a paper in your right hand, fold it in half, and put it on the floor); Ask the patient to write a sentence (note handedness in writing) or to copy a simple design; Patient's ability to follow and execute the previous requests; Possibility of dominant hemisphere language impairment, i.e., aphasia, dysarthria, etc. Note whether patient or family members have left handedness or history of learning disability)

E. *Abstract Thinking:* (Ability to abstract and generalize. Proverbs interpretation; Similarities; Differences; Essence or moral of small story, etc.)

F. *General Fund of Information and Awareness of Current Events:* (Include awareness of current events in the context of patient's social-educational background, e.g., Who is the President of the United States, etc.)

G. *Insight:* (Degree of awareness and understanding by the patient of his illness and situation. Complete denial of illness; Slight awareness of being sick and needing help but denying it at the same time; Awareness of being sick but blaming it on others or on external factors; Recognition of the illness and acceptance of treatment)

H. *Judgement:* (Social judgement. Does the patient understand the likely outcome of his behavior and is he influenced by this understanding. Test judgement. Ask patient what he would do if he finds an envelope in the street that is sealed, addressed, and has a new stamp or if, while in the movies, he is the first person to see smoke and fire)

I. *Intelligence:* (Results of most recent psychometric testing, i.e., Full Scale IQ, name of test, year; If unavailable, give your clinical impression based on the current Cognitive Functions Examination — Retarded, Average range, Low Average range, High Average range, etc.)

II. DIAGNOSIS

DSM III-R Diagnosis According to Axes I-V
(Indicate PRINCIPAL DIAGNOSIS by an "X" in the appropriate "O"
CHECK EITHER AXIS I OR AXIS II—NEVER BOTH)
Axis I—Clinical Syndromes and V Codes
_____._____ O

_____._____

_____._____
Axis II—Developmental Disorder and Personality Disorders
_____._____ O

_____._____

_____._____
Axis III—Physical Disorders and Conditions (ICD-9-CM Codes)
_____._____

_____._____

_____._____
Axis IV—Severity of Psychosocial Stressors
Stressor(s):
Severity (Check one):
1. None 2. Mild 3. Moderate 4. Severe 5. Extreme
6. Catastrophic
0. Inadequate information or no change in condition

Duration (Check one):
_____ Predominantly Acute Event
_____ Predominantly Enduring Circumstances
Axis V—Global Assessment of Functioning
(Enter two digit scores from 01-90)
_____ Current GAF score (the level of functioning at the time of evaluation)
_____ Past Year GAF (the highest level of functioning for at least a few months during the past year. For children and adolescents this must include at least a month during the school year

III. ASSESSMENT AND PROGNOSIS

1. *PSYCHIATRIC PROBLEMS:* (Intellectual, Cognitive, Emotional and Behavioral Dysfunctions and Disorders which are focus of treatment. Key issue here is focus of treatment. Limit specific problems

(product of symptoms, character, and personality) to those which are keeping the patient in the hospital/clinic or at current level of care, which can be reasonably expected to improve with proper and consistent application of treatment (methods). Prioritize these problems in the context of the expected next level of least restrictive care, i.e., pass card, open ward setting, discharge, etc. Patient may have many problems but some must be treated and resolved first, before others can be addressed. Describe behaviorally, without unnecessary historical detail (which is available in the assessment) and without using psychiatric terminology (such as delusional, hallucinating, strong dependency needs, poor impulse control, etc.). Group together behavioral problems which are either etiologically or otherwise related to each other, e.g., refusal to take medications, physical examinations are usually part of paranoid behavior or syndrome)

2. *PHYSICAL/MEDICAL PROBLEMS:* (Use legend above as appropriate)

3. *STRENGTHS:* (Identify strengths/assets which are directly related to the above psychiatric and physical (medical) problems and could be used to enhance treatment (methods). Describe them behaviorally as in problems. Avoid the use of terms such as "cooperative, ambulatory" and other non-specific or unrelated terms)

4. *DISABILITIES:* (Longstanding impairments, often irreversible, which may interfere with the focus of treatment or adequate functions generally. Specify physical/medical issues which alter or preclude treatment methods or render the problem untreatable at this time. Keep the disabilities that are current)

5. *PROGNOSIS:* (Opinion as to the probable future course, extent, and outcome of the illness. Give reasons for a certain prognosis based not only on natural history of illness, but also characterological and environmental factors such as insight, non-compliance, poor response to treatment, alcohol/substance abuse, non-supportive or absent family, lack of financial resources, poor education, poor vocational skills and work history, poor interpersonal and social skills, poor adaptation in placement settings, etc.)

IV. *TREATMENT RECOMMENDATIONS:* (Should be based on identified, treatable problems that have specific strengths to address them and are not seriously compromised by a disability)

1. *PSYCHOPHARMACOLOGICAL TREATMENT:* (Identify psychopharmacological agents by group for specific symptoms such as anti-psychotics, anti-depressants, etc. Dosage range. Serum levels. Any initial laboratory work up needed. Follow up and monitoring plans. Plans for psychopharmacological consultations; Internal or external case reviews; Referral to Movement Disorder Clinic, etc.)

2. *MEDICAL TREATMENTS:* (Follow the legend as noted above. Most of the information should be available in the current physical assessment)

3. *OTHER TREATMENTS:* (Include any other interventions or recommendations such as individual therapy, group therapy, activities therapy, workshop, pass card, etc., for specific problems)

4. *ALLERGIES/SENSITIVITIES:* (Allergies to drugs or other substances; Sensitivity to certain drugs)

V. *PHYSICIAN OR PSYCHIATRIST SIGNATURE, TITLE, AND DATE*

APPENDIX B

CORE HISTORY Rev. 6/9/91

ROCKLAND PSYCHIATRIC CENTER

C O R E   H I S T O R Y

INSTRUCTIONS:
—Initiate on first contact or admission but must complete by the due date of first treatment plan meeting.
—Completed by social worker; reviewed and co-signed by psychiatrist.
—Update continuously during the course of treatment as significant life events occur or additional data becomes available. Use continuation sheets.

Patient Data: Lastname, Firstname, MI
                     C#, DOB
                     Unit/Ward, Sex

1. *SOURCE OF INFORMATION and RELIABILITY:* (Indicate the person(s) providing the information, such as patient, member of the fam-

ily, previous medical records, records from other hospitals, etc., and estimate of reliability of the information provided)

2. *CURRENT LEGAL STATUS:* (If involuntary/court retained give date of expiration)

3. *IDENTIFYING DATA:*

3A. (Include Age (Date of Birth); Marital Status; Race/ethnicity; Sex; Religion; Date of Admission/Transfer, referral source; Admission/ transfer Legal Status; Means of transportation; Name, relationship, and phone number of individual(s) who accompanied the patient)

3B. *OTHER INFORMATION:*
1. Maiden name or A.K.A.:
2. Primary language:
3. Address on admission:
4. County of Residence:
5. Education:
6. Veteran Status:
7. Prior State Facility/State I.D. No.:
8. Social Security No.:
9. Medicare No.:
10. Medicaid No.:
11. Other Health Insurance and Number:
12. 620/621 Eligible:

4. *REASONS FOR CURRENT ADMISSION:* (Chronological background and development of symptoms or behavioral changes leading up to this admission; Life circumstances at the time of onset of the current illness, how illness affected activities, personal and family relationships, work and leisure activities; Duration of current illness and disabilities the illness produced. Include patient's chief complaints in his/her words with any precipitating factors; include any reports or complaints from family, friends and any other people or agencies. Any treatment patient is receiving and at what clinic or privately; include the name of the psychiatrist, names and dosage of medications and when and what medications were taken last time)

5. *PERSONAL DEVELOPMENTAL HISTORY—ANAMNESIS:* (History of the patient's life from infancy to the current hospitalization, including information regarding birth, developmental milestones, adjustment or behavioral disturbances during childhood, adolescence, and

adulthood, school adjustments, educational history, highest educational status achieved, military, occupational and vocational history, psychosexual history, marital history, any children and any history of mental illness or alcohol/substance abuse in them, any unusual illness)

6. *LIVING ARRANGEMENT:* (Include with whom the patient lives; housing pattern/stability, and desire and ability to return)

7. *USE OF LEISURE TIME:* (Include patient's hobbies and other activities which he/she enjoys)

8. *PAST PSYCHIATRIC HISTORY:* (Age at onset of the illness: Chronological background and development of symptoms or behavioral changes leading to first treatment and/or hospitalization, including nature (clinical features) of illness; Life circumstances at the time of onset of illness and its effect on activities and personal relationships; Dates of previous hospitalizations; Names of the hospitals; Circumstances of hospitalizations; Treatments prescribed and their effects; Discharges and aftercare plans; Reasons for the failure of these discharges or placements; Medications on discharge issues of compliance with aftercare plans)

9. *PAST DISCHARGE/PLACEMENT HISTORY:* (Describe in chronological order all previous discharges/placements until the time of this admission. Include the name and types of placements, i.e., pt.'s family, S.R.O., P.P.H.A., Family Care Home, R.C.C.A., S.O.C.C.A., etc. Other aftercare plans including the name of the mental health clinic. Duration of each placement and reasons for failure)

10. *ALCOHOL/SUBSTANCE ABUSE HISTORY:* (Pattern of abuse; Alcohol/Substance seeking behavior, its effect on work, relationships, problems with the law, arrests, imprisonments, etc.; Any treatment received for these problems including residential and outpatient)

11. *LEGAL HISTORY:* (History of any arrests, imprisonments, current legal issues, charges, CPL status, etc.)

12. *FAMILY HISTORY:* (Family background, financial, educational, religious, and vocational status of parents; Number of siblings; Relationship of the pt. with family of origin; History of mental illness, and alcohol/substance abuse and diagnosis of these illnesses in the family,

history of psychiatric hospitalization and medication history if applicable and available; Relevant family medical history)

13. *MEDICAL HISTORY:* (Include past and current medical history. Medical diagnosis, medications and others treatments, the name of medications, doses, name, address and phone number of the physician(s). Include the date of last contact with family physician and, if applicable, gynecologist)

14. *ALLERGIES/SENSITIVITIES:* (Include any allergies and sensitivities to any particular medications)

15. *BURIAL INFORMATION/PLOT/FUNDS:* ONLY IF RELEVANT, UPDATE AS INDICATED. (Describe whether pt. has any burial funds, amount; Bank account; Burial plot, deed, location, etc.)

Completed by: _____   Date: _____
                    Team Social Worker

Reviewed by: _____   Date: _____
                    Team Psychiatrist

APPENDIX C

DISCHARGE SUMMARY Rev. 6/29/91

ROCKLAND PSYCHIATRIC CENTER

DISCHARGE SUMMARY

INSTRUCTIONS:
    — Initiate few days before discharge but must complete within one week of the date of discharge.
    — Review Core History, Social and Psychiatric Assessments. Include only pertinent information as indicated.
    — Focus on treatment course and recommendations for the after care clinic staff and other providers.

Patient Data: Lastname, Firstname, MI
                         C#, DOB
                         Unit/Ward, Sex

1. *IDENTIFYING DATA:* (Include Age (Date of Birth); Marital Status; Race/ethnicity; Sex; Religion; Date of Admission/Transfer, from where; Admission/transfer Legal Status; Means of transportation; Name, relationship, and phone number of individual(s) who accompanied the patient.)

2. *REASONS FOR CURRENT ADMISSION:* (Chronological background and development of symptoms or behavioral changes leading up to this admission; Life circumstances at the time of onset of the current illness, how illness affected activities, personal and family relationships, work and leisure activities; Duration of current illness and disabilities the illness produced. Include patient's chief complaints in his/her words with any precipitating factors; include any reports or complaints from family, friends and any other people or agencies. Any treatment patient is receiving and at what clinic or privately; include the name of the psychiatrist, names and dosage of medications and when and what medications were taken last time.)

3. *ADMISSION DIAGNOSIS:*

Axis I:
Axis II:
Axis III:
Axis IV:
Axis V: GAF Score:

4. *FAMILY HISTORY:* (Family background, financial, educational, religious, and vocational status of parents; Number of siblings; Relationship of the pt. with family of origin; History of mental illness, and alcohol/substance abuse and diagnosis of these illnesses in the family, history of psychiatric hospitalization and medication history if applicable and available; Relevant family medical history.)

5. *PERSONAL DEVELOPMENTAL HISTORY–ANAMNESIS:* (History of the patient's life from infancy to the current hospitalization, including information regarding birth, developmental milestones, adjustment or behavioral disturbances during childhood, adolescence and adulthood, school adjustments, educational history, highest educational status achieved, military and occupational, vocational history, psychosexual history, marital history, any children and any mental illness or alcohol/substance abuse history in them, any unusual illness.)

6. *PAST PSYCHIATRIC HISTORY:* (Age at onset of the illness; Chronological background and development of symptoms or behavioral changes leading to first treatment and/or hospitalization, including nature (clinical features) of illness; Life circumstances at the time of onset of illness and its effect on activities and personal relationships; Dates of previous hospitalizations; Names of the hospitals; Circumstances of hospitalizations; Treatments prescribed and their effects; Discharges and aftercare plans; Reasons for the failure of these discharges or placements; Medications on discharge issues of compliance with aftercare plans.)

7. *ALCOHOL/SUBSTANCE ABUSE HISTORY:* (Pattern of abuse; Alcohol/Substance seeking behavior, its effect on work, relationships, problems with the law, arrests, imprisonments, etc.; Any treatment received for these problems including residential and outpatient.)

8. *PSYCHIATRIC TREATMENT COURSE:* (Summary of the psychiatric treatment course from the date of admission to the date of discharge and or termination. Summarize the previous treatment course in Psychiatric assessments. Focus on main psychiatric and behavioral problems on admission and subsequent changes with treatment. Include specific problems such as assaultiveness, suicidal or homicidal behavior, elopement, etc. Use of restraint or seclusion, PRN medications, duration of these problem behaviors modifications and or improvements. Specify last incident of such behaviors. Summarize the psychopharmacological interventions and its rationale, including the name of the drugs, dosage, effects, side-effects and any sensitivities. Include last serum level reports with dates. Your opinion as to the best regimen and its rationale; Summarize other psycho-social interventions used such as individual, group, and family psychotherapies, their rationale and outcome. Use of pass card, home leaves, level of contact and availability of family members or significant others. Patient's level of involvement in rehabilitative and vocational activities. Summarize any special testing done such as psychometric evaluation, vocational, educational, and other assessments, including diagnostic impressions, recommendations and its outcome. (If relevant, include the circumstances of patient's death, diagnosis, autopsy results and other relevant data.)

9. *MEDICAL TREATMENT COURSE:* (Summary of physical/medical treatment course from the date of admission to the date of discharge and or termination. Include the date of last physical examination and

its findings. Include abnormal findings of the various laboratory workups including the dates of the last reports. Review various specialty consultations made, diagnosis, recommendations, and followup. Include allergies and or sensitivities.)

10. *CURRENT MENTAL STATUS EXAMINATION:* (Brief version of all the items in Mental Status Exam from Psychiatric Assessment.)

11. *FINAL FUNCTIONAL ASSESSMENT:* (Include in summary form how the patient is functioning now; Degree of remission (full, partial). Be descriptive in discussing strengths and assets which could be used to enhance treatment provided by psychiatrist and other aftercare providers, as well as problems which may be encountered.)

12. *FINAL DIAGNOSIS:*

Axis I:
Axis II:
Axis III:
GAF Score:

13. *AFTERCARE PLANS:*

1. *LIVING ARRANGEMENT:* (Where patient will be residing. Type of place, e.g., patient's family, own home, family care home, P.P.H.A., R.C.C.A., S.O.C.A.R. etc., Suggestions for the staff and or provider to deal with anticipated problems.)

2. *PSYCHIATRIC FOLLOW-UP:* (Include name of the M.H.C. and or the private practitioner; its address and phone number, and the date of first appointment.)

3. *MEDICAL FOLLOW-UP:* (Include physical health care needs. Name of the physician, office address, and telephone number; Date of appointment.)

4. *MEDICATIONS AND SUPPLY ON DISCHARGE:* (Include each medication separately, dosage and total days of supply.)

5. *CASE MANAGER STATUS, (IF APPLICABLE):* (Include the name of the case manager, address, and phone number and any other pertinent information.)

14. *SIGNATURE, TITLE, AND DATE:*

Tickler:
An Automated System
to Monitor Assessment Dates
for Psychiatric Care

Anjan Bhattacharyya

KEYWORDS. Computerized medical record, medical record reminder system, mental health software, computerized quality assurance system

PROBLEM SCENARIO

The setting for this study is an inpatient treatment unit in a state operated psychiatric care facility treating 250 patients with acute and chronic psychiatric symptomatology. A basic team of psychiatrists together with social workers, psychologists and a secretary interacts to provide proper clinical care. Each patient needs at least twelve different types of assessments at different days in a year. Each assessment has its own characteristics and complexities. The clinical assessments require varieties of professional expertise, but problems are encountered in *knowing who is scheduled and when* and *what type of assessment is needed, and for which patients, and by which clinicians*. The traditional method of depending on a secretary or other administrative staff member to inform the clinician is very confusing, and less reliable. This scheduling limitation is being experienced as a significant detriment to the delivery of timely clinical care.

Anjan Bhattacharyya is Director of the Microcomputing Department, Quality Assurance Division, at Rockland Psychiatric Center, Orangeburg, NY 10962.

MOTIVATION FOR AN AUTOMATED SYSTEM

The scheduling problem has multiple variables. Traditional methods of handling this involves laborious hand written lists and data collection which are monotonous and subject to greater human error. The incentive to develop this application started with the hope of reducing an error prone, non-systematic method of day to day scheduling, improving the efficiency of administering our clinical information system, and providing better clinical care by providing information quickly and accurately.

The chaos encountered by the clinical staff members on a daily basis to find out who is scheduled and when and for what services was incredibly long and tedious and many times inaccurate. The process was using up much of the clinicians' available time. This type of paperwork chaos is not new or unique to our hospital. In any facility, where the staff resources are limited, clinicians devote much time in performing the administrative paperwork just to find out what tasks need to be done and for what purpose. With the ever increasing demand of regulatory agencies and quality of care regulations, management of such basic scheduling information becomes an almost unbearable burden, one which is enjoyed by very few clinicians. This task gets more complicated in any dynamic environment where the patient turnover is high and where the turnover of clinical staff members may also be high.

Since one of the major controlling components of clinical care is the *date* (a fundamental piece of data to monitor any aspect of care) we focused on using the date as a major primary key. The clinical care team felt that it would be an excellent support to have a profile on each patient with various treatment dates, listing when each treatment was due and when it was accomplished. After a preliminary systems analysis, it became obvious that a database application program would be necessary to resolve this problem.

WHAT IS A TICKLER

The Tickler System is an application program developed for the purpose of monitoring all the *assessment dates* for various types of treatment services rendered to the patients residing at the Rockland

Psychiatric Center. The application program developed with the goals of minimum data input to generate maximum output in the desired report forms. Its user friendliness is accomplished with a carefully designed menu system. We called it a TICKLER since it reminds the clinicians on a daily basis about the scheduling of patients to receive assessment and treatment.

The system design of the TICKLER was defined on the basis of tasks to maintain very basic goals of monitoring a patient list and assessment schedule date list. Thus, the fundamental functional items such as add, edit, delete and print features were incorporated for both the databases. After outlining the basic goals of the project was written down, the designing of the database structure began.

The *TICKLER* program interfaces with two different databases. They are, Patient Database and, Assessment Scheduling database. The Patient Database contains the all necessary administrative, demographic, and some clinical information. The variables included in Patient Database system are as follows:

> patient last name, patient first name, consecutive number, unit code, ward, admission date, date of birth, sex, race, physician, team leader, social worker.

The Assessment Scheduling database contains a list of all the assessments and the last date of completion for each assessment. The Assessment Scheduling database can only be invoked with a correct consecutive number in the Patient Database. Thus, the system will not allow any data in the Assessment Scheduling Database system without patient information in the Patient Database system. Once the assessment completion date is entered in the system, *TICKLER* will automatically compute the *next due date*, as well as the *over due date* for each assessment as of the current or system date. The data structures included in Assessment Scheduling Database system are the *dates of services* of the following:

> comprehensive assessment, laboratory assessment, physical examination, physical assessment, psychiatric assessment, nutritional assessment, psychological assessment, quarterly review, nursing assessment, social assessment, activity assessment, educational assessment, vocational assessment,

periodic review date for newly admitted and age under 22 years of age.

Two customized forms were developed to gather patient and assessment information. The TICKLER system prevents duplicate patient numbers and various sorts of assessments dates. A message informs a user if duplicate information is entered.

IMPLEMENTATION

The TICKLER system is designed to be used in a computer with DOS environment along with the software called R:BASE for DOS. The installation of this application software is very straightforward. The coded files are written in R:Base programming language, and is stored in a subdirectory within the R:Base application subdirectory. This application can be invoked by typing TICKLER at the DOS C prompt. It is important to note that organization of these application files and other file management issues can be custom designed to suit the users' need and individual hardware configuration. The effectiveness of the memory management and speed is improved when this application is run on a computer with hard disk and RAM of at least 640K.

FEATURES

This application is written on the foundation of structured programming. This modularity allows better upgrading of the system to accommodate users' specific needs and requirements. Access to data as well as report generation can be protected with a password protection scheme. The original data structure can be protected from novice users for any inadvertent changes. The most interesting feature of this application, (once the user has learned some basis knowledge of using R:Base) is that the user has the option of generating unique reports, if not satisfied with canned report forms, thus improving the versatility.

To reduce input keystroke errors, TICKLER is rule based on certain fields such as patients name [upper case only] and consecutive number. The application first requires pertinent information on the

Patient Database prior to processing information on Assessment Due Database. For the assessment date database, the application is designed in such a way that it is not necessary to input any other information of a patient except the consecutive number. The assessment scheduling database will not be activated unless the consecutive number is current in the patient database. This feature has significantly improved the data integrity. It computes the virtual due date on any assessment based on a predetermined formula which is established by the facility administrator, outside regulatory agencies, or internal medical staff organization.

Once the servicing unit is organized and trained to use this application, it requires very little time [less than a minute per record to input] for an average user to perform the I/O operation. The learning curve for this application is very rapid.

LIMITATION

Most users want a computer application, which is compiled and executable at the DOS prompt since this is more simple and faster. Unfortunately, this application is not compiled (in its current version) and is not executable so that it can run directly from DOS. It would be possible to compile the R:Base language in this application so that any user could use it without a copy of R:Base software. The current version will run somewhat slower than would the compiled version.

REPORTS

Several standard reports are included in the menu. The application also has the capability to generate any custom reports not included in the menu mode. The pilot testing of this application had an astounding success, improving enormous amount of clinical care time and providing documentation on appropriate clinical service records on assigned patients. Fourteen different canned reports are included in this application. It was found sufficient to cover a broad spectrum of treatment care. Sample reports are attached in the appendix.

SUMMARY

This system provided us with tangible benefits of rapid scheduling and information retrieval. We are less dependent on specific personnel. This has reduced error in the clinical information system. It provided the administrator with improved efficiency in the management of clinician time. We are now more prepared for inspection by our regulatory agencies at all times. The TICKLER has been found to be a very fruitful workhorse with efficiency. Anxiety about compliance with required reports is reduced and a big headache is reduced to pleasure. The clinician-computer interaction became quicker (and friendlier) as the use of computer increased.

PROSPECT FOR FURTHER UPGRADING

Because of the modularity of design, the application can be easily accommodated into other programs that might be developed at a later date. An experienced user can get into the R:Base R > prompt and use the database to generate various other reports that are not available in the application. If necessary, the user can add other variables to expand the database and satisfy user-specific needs. During the writing of this paper, our current system got updated with several new features, illustrating the flexibility and modularity of the design.

SOFTWARE AVAILABILITY

The source code for the TICKLER is included in the APPENDIX and is also available on the TESTING STATION BBS (see Chapter 2).

REFERENCE

R:BASE for DOS, Version 2.11 (1989). Redmond, Washington, Microrim Corporation.

APPENDIX A: INSTALLATION INSTRUCTION

1] Install R:base for DOS following software instructions
2] Make a subdirectory called TICKLER on your hard drive within DBFILES subdirectory as shown below:

MD C:/DBFILES/TICKLER [enter]

3] Follow instruction to copy the application in your hard drive in the path of C:/DBFILES/TICKLER:

COPY A:/DBFILES/TICKLER/*.* C:/DBFILES/TICKLER

4] Invoke the application by typing TICKLER at the C:
5] Follow the menu driven system. The application includes a couple of demo records for your review.

APPENDIX B: MENU SCREEN

PATIENT TICKLER SYSTEM

(1) PATIENT DATA
(2) SCHEDULE DATA
(3) GENERATE SCHEDULE REPORTS
(4) PERFORM BACKUP – PLACE FORMATTED DISK IN DRIVE "A"
(5) EXIT – BACKUP ALL CHANGES BEFORE EXITING THIS PROGRAM

APPENDIX B: MENU SCREEN

PATIENT DATA

(1) ADD PATIENT
(2) EDIT/BROWSE/DELETE
(3) EXIT BACK TO MAIN PROGRAM

APPENDIX B: MENU SCREEN

CHOOSE REPORT

(1) COMBINED ASSESSMENT REPORT
(2) EDUCATIONAL ASSESSMENT REPORT

(3) LABORATORY ROUTINE REPORT
(4) PATIENT CARE ASSESSMENT REPORT
(5) NUTRITIONAL ASSESSMENT REPORT
(6) PATIENT DATA REPORT (USE 15CPI FONT IN 8.5" BY 11"
  PAPER)
(7) PSYCHIATRIC ASSESSMENT
(8) MORE REPORTS
(9) EXIT TO MAIN PROGRAM

Select Print Routing

Printer   Screen   Both

APPENDIX C: MENU SCREEN

ADDITIONAL ASSESSMENT REPORT

(1) PHYSICAL ASSESSMENT REPORT
(2) PHYSICAL EXAMINATION REPORT
(3) QUARTERLY REVIEW REPORT
(4) SOCIAL ASSESSMENT REPORT
(5) VOCATIONAL ASSESSMENT REPORT
(6) ACTIVITY ASSESSMENT REPORT
(7) EXIT TO MAIN PROGRAM

Select Print Routing

Printer   Screen   Both

APPENDIX C: INPUT SCREEN

Add   Duplicate   Edit again   Discard   Quit

PATIENT DATA INPUT FORM

PATIENT LAST NAME :
PATIENT FIRST NAME   :
CONSECUTIVE NUMBER   :
UNIT CODE   :
WARD   :
ADMISSION DATE   :
DATE OF BIRTH   :

                  SEX   :
                  RACE   :
                  PHYSICIAN   :
                  TEAM LEADER   :
                  SOCIAL WORKER   :

[Esc] Done [F2] Clear field [Shift-F2] Clear to end [Shift-F10] More
Form: PTDATA *Table*: PTDATA *Field*: LNAME *Page*: 1

APPENDIX C: INPUT SCREEN

Add   Duplicate   Edit again   Discard   Quit

ASSESSMENT SCHEDULING FORM
ENTER DATE COMPLETED FOR EACH ASSESSMENT

          PATIENT LAST NAME   :
          PATIENT FIRST NAME   :
          CONSECUTIVE NUMBER   :
          UNIT CODE   :
          COMPREHENSIVE DATE   :
          LABORATORY ASSESSMENT DATE   :
          PHYSICAL EXAMINATION DATE   :
          PHYSICAL ASSESSMENT DATE   :
          PSYCHIATRIC ASSESSMENT DATE   :
          NUTRITIONAL ASSESSMENT DATE   :
          PSYCHOLOGICAL ASSESSMENT DATE   : .
          QUARTERLY REVIEW DATE   :
          NURSING ASSESSMENT DATE   :
          SOCIAL ASSESSMENT DATE   :
          ACTIVITY ASSESSMENT DATE   :
          EDUCATIONAL ASSESSMENT DATE   :
          VOCATIONAL ASSESSMENT DATE   :

[Esc] Done [F2] Clear field [Shift-F2] Clear to end [Shift-F10] More
Form: PTSCHED *Table:* PTSCHED *Field:* LNAME Page: 1

APPENDIX D: INSTRUCTION MANUAL

TO ACCESS AND RUN TICKLER APPLICATION:
* Turn on the computer by flipping up the start switch,
* Type TICKLER at C: prompt
  then, press the Enter key.
* The Patient Tickler System Menu will appear on the screen with the following options:
  - (1) PATIENT DATA
  - (2) SCHEDULE DATA
  - (3) GENERATE SCHEDULE REPORTS
  - (4) PERFORM BACKUP
  - (5) EXIT
* Select your option by typing the corresponding number and press the Enter key.

(1) PATIENT DATA:
* To get access to the PATIENT DATA File, Select option (1) from PATIENT TICKLER SYSTEM Menu and press the Enter Key.
* The PATIENT DATA Menu will appear on the screen with the following options:
  - (1) ADD PATIENT
  - (2) EDIT/BROWSE/DELETE
  - (3) EXIT
* Select your choice by typing the choice number and press the Enter key.

ADD PATIENT
* To add a new record to the Patient Data File, highlight the ADD PATIENT option or Type 1 and press the Enter key.
* A Patient Data Input Form will appear on the screen, as shown in the input screen.
* Type in the data that you wish to store.
* Press the Enter key after typing each field to store the data, and to move to the next field.
* When you finish typing a patient record, press the Enter key. A menu appears across the top of the screen with the following options:

Add:　　　　adds the data you just entered and prepares screen for next entry.

Duplicate:　adds the data, but leaves it on the screen so it may be edited. This is useful only if there are slight differences between successive entries.

Edit again: edit data you just entered.
Discard: removes data and allow you to start again.
Quit: ends the entry, like pressing <Esc>.

- Highlight the appropriate command.
- Type in the data of the new record, field by field.
- After completion of the data entry, press Esc key to get back to the PATIENT DATA MENU. This may have to be done twice.
  EDIT/BROWSE/DELETE:
- EDIT means to make a change in the PATIENT DATA BASE entry.
- BROWSE means displays data while scrolling up, down, left and right in the rows and columns of a table.
- DELETE means to delete a record from a table or a field from a record.
- To EDIT/BROWSE/DELETE a PATIENT DATA ENTRY, highlight option 2 from the PATIENT DATA MENU and press ENTER KEY.
- The edit screen will display all patient data in alphabetical order by last name, unit and ward.
- Move the highlighting to the column you need to edit by pressing the TAB key to move to the right or press Shift and Tab keys simultaneously to move to the left.
- After you make your corrections in a record, press Up or Down arrow keys to move to another record.
- If, while editing a single field of data, you find that you've made a mistake, you can "undo" your edit as long as the highlight is still on the same field.
- To restore the original contents to the field being edited, press the F5 key on the keyboard.
- To DELETE a row (record) from the DATA BASE while the edit screen is showing, use the up and down arrow keys to move the highlighting to the row that you want to delete.
- When that row is highlighted, press the F2 key.
- Press Enter to delete the row or press Esc to change your mind.
- When done with all the editing procedures, press Escape Key to get back to the PATIENT DATA MENU.
  EXIT
- You have now added some records to the PATIENT DATA BASE by using ADD DATA option.
- You've edited (changed) some items of information using the EDIT/ BROWSE/DELETE option from PATIENT DATE MENU.

- You want to get back to PATIENT TICKLER SYSTEM, by moving the highlight to the EXIT option on the PATIENT DATA MENU, and press Enter.
- You are back to the PATIENT TICKLER SYSTEM MENU with its Five options:

> (1) PATIENT DATA
> (2) SCHEDULE DATA
> (3) GENERATE SCHEDULE REPORTS
> (4) PERFORM BACKUP(5) EXIT

(2) SCHEDULE DATA

- If you select Schedule Data option 2, and press Enter Key you will get to the Assessment Schedules Menu with the following options:

> 1. ENTER SCHEDULES
> 2. EDIT/BROWSE/DELETE
> 3. EXIT

ENTER SCHEDULES

- Type 1, and press the Enter Key to select ENTER SCHEDULES option.
- An ASSESSMENT SCHEDULING FORM will be shown on the screen as shown in input screen.
- Enter the date of completion for each assessment.
- Press the Enter Key after each entry to store the data.
- Any assessment schedule data entered into the ASSESSMENT SCHEDULE FORM must contain a correctly spelled patient name and consecutive number that exists in the PATIENT DATA file. Otherwise, the schedule data will be rejected and the error message : "CHECK DATA ENTRY IN PATIENT DATA" will appear on the top of the screen.
- To check the DATA ENTRY in PATIENT DATA:

1. Press ESC, an options menu will appear across the top of the screen
2. Highlight <Discard> key using the arrow keys.
3. Press Enter key twice to discard entry.
4. Press Esc key three times to return to "TICKLER."
5. Highlight (1) Patient Data and press Enter.
6. Highlight (2) Edit/Browse/Delete and press Enter key.
7. Follow Editing Procedures to locate patient.
8. Correct spelling.

9. If patient is not listed, then NO schedules can be entered until the patient data are entered. Press Esc and either enter patient data or press Esc again to return to schedules.

• After you done with all your entries, Press ESC for the following menu options:

[Add, Duplicate, Edit again, Discard, Quit].

• Highlight the Quit option to get back to the ASSESSMENT SCHEDULING MENU with the following options:

1. ENTER SCHEDULES
2. EDIT/BROWSE/DELETE
3. EXIT

EDIT/BROWSE/DELETE
• Select option 2, to get access to the EDIT/BROWSE/DELETE option.
• Follow the EDIT/BROWSE/DELETE Procedures as previously explained in the PATIENT DATA.
• After the completion of the editing procedures, press ESC key to go back to the ASSESSMENT SCHEDULES Menu.
• Select EXIT option, to go back to PATIENT TICKLER SYSTEM Menu.

(3) GENERATE SCHEDULE REPORTS

• Select option 3, for Generate Schedule Reports menu and press Enter key, a list of assessment Reports will appear on the screen for your choice.
1. Combined Assessment
2. Educational Assessment
3. Laboratory Routine Reports
4. Patient Care Assessment
5. Nutritional Assessment
6. Psychiatric Assessment
7. Physical Assessment
8. Physical Examination
9. Quarterly Review
10. Social Assessment
11. Vocational Assessment
12. Activity Assessment

- Select the report of Your choice by typing the number, and press the Enter Key.
- For example, If you choose report (1), type 1, and press Enter, a select print routing menu will appear on the screen with three choices: (printer, screen, both).
- Make your choice for the output format by moving the cursor with the arrow keys, and then press the Enter key.
- If you select <screen>, the scrolling display may be halted by pressing the Pause key. Scrolling will begin again by pressing any key.
- When you finish with your reports, press the Esc key twice get back to the patient tickler system.
- To exit from tickler system press the Esc key. This will take you back to the R > prompt.
- To leave R Base, type exit and press the Enter Key.
- Other reports can be generated as needed by any sorting orders.

(4) PERFORM BACKUP

It is important to have a duplicate copy of your data. To save a copy of the most current data, first make a formatted disk and then keep it in drive A, before your press the number (4) in the PATIENT TICK-LER SYSTEM.

(5) EXIT

- Use exit option and hit the Enter key, it will bring it back to DOS C prompt.
- When you finish with your final work, press number 5 to get to R > prompt.
- To leave R Base, type exit and press the Enter Key.

APPENDIX E: EXAMPLES OF SAMPLE REPORTS

TYPE: 1

LISTING OF PATEINTS DEMOGRAPHIC PROFILE BY WARD
AS OF 04/16/91

WARD	PATIENT NAME	CNO	AGE	SEX	RACE
11	Robert Roberts	123	45	m	b
11	Jimmy Jones	321	54	m	w
11	Pat Cucumber	345	32	f	w
*******************					
172	Richard Richardson	987	27	m	w
172	Donald Dunkings	789	53	m	b

TYPE: 2   PAGE 1

COMPREHENSIVE ASSESSMENT DATES
AS OF 04/16/91

PATIENT NAME + DUE	CONSEC#	ADM DATE	DATE DONE	DATE DUE	WARD	
Robert Roberts	123	07/15/86	-0-	-0-	11	-0-
Jimmy Jones	321	07/31/87	05/20/89	05/11/90	11	341
Pat Cucumber	345	07/15/86	-0-	-0-	11	-0-
********************						
Richard Richardson	987	12/02/85	02/23/89	02/24/90	172	417
Donald Dunkings	789	04/27/49	10/08/88	10/09/89	172	555

TYPE: 3
                                                                          PAGE 1

LISTING OF PATIENT ASSESSMENT DUE DATES BY WARD
AS OF 04/16/91

PATIENT NAME	CONSEC#	COMPDUE	PXDUE	PSYDUE
Robert Roberts	123	03/13/90	03/09/90	04/13/90
Jimmy Jones	321	05/31/90	09/21/89	10/25/89
Pat Cucumber	345	06/17/90	05/24/90	03/29/90
******************				
Richard Richardson	987	07/28/89	12/20/89	12/02/89
Donald Dunkings	789	11/28/89	05/19/90	05/29/89

TYPE: 4

LISTING OF PATIENTS CLINICAL INFORMATION BY WARD
AS OF 04/16/91

WARD TEAM LEADER	PATIENT NAME	ADM DATE	LOS	PHYSICIAN	
11	Robert Roberts	07/15/86	1146	KLOTH	DeVIVO
11	Jimmy Jones	07/31/87	781	KUNDU	CHIANG
11	Pat Cucumber	07/15/86	1162	OEI	GERMANO
•••••••••••••••••••					
172	Richard Richardson	12/02/85	470	WINTERS	BULLOCK
172	Donald Dunkings	04/27/49	•755	WINTERS	BULLOCK

TYPE: 5

PAGE 1

QAURTERLY REVIEW DATES
AS OF 04/16/91

PATIENT NAME	CONSEC#	ADN DATE	DATE DONE	DATE DUE	WARD	+ DUE
Robert Roberts	123	07/15/86	-0-	-0-	11	-0-
Jimmy Jones	321	07/31/87	05/23/89	08/22/89	11	602
Pat Cucumber	345	07/15/86	-0-	-0-	11	-0-
•••••••••••••••••						
Richard Richardson	987	12/02/85	02/23/89	02/24/90	172	417
Donald Dunkings	789	04/27/49	10/08/88	10/09/89	172	555

TYPE: 6

PAGE 1

ACTIVITY ASSESSMENT DATES
AS OF 04/16/91

PATIENT NAME	CONSEC#	ADM DATE	DATE DONE	DATE DUE	WARD	+ DUE
Robert Roberts	123	07/15/86	-0-	-0-	11	-0-
Jimmy Jones	321	07/31/87	05/20/89	05/11/90	11	341
Pat Cucumber	345	07/15/86	-0-	-0-	11	-0-
•••••••••••••••••						
Richard Richardson	987	12/02/85	02/23/90	172	417	
Donald Dunkings	789	04/27/49	10/08/88	10/09/89	172	555

APPENDIX F: SOURCE CODE FOR TICKLER

```
$COMMAND
TICKLER
SET MESSAGE OFF
OPEN SCHED
SET ERROR MESSAGE OFF
SET COLOR BACKGRND BLUE
SET COLOR FOREGRND WHITE
SET BELL OFF
SET VAR PICK1 INT
LABEL STARTAPP
  NEWPAGE
  CHOOSE PICK1 FROM Main IN TICKLER.Apx
  IF PICK1 EQ 1 THENSET VAR PICK2 INT
    SET VAR LEVEL2 INT
    SET VAR LEVEL2 TO 0
    WHILE LEVEL2 EQ 0 THEN
      NEWPAGE
      CHOOSE PICK2 FROM INPUT IN TICKLER.Apx
      IF PICK2 EQ 0 THEN
        BREAK
      ENDIF
      IF PICK2 EQ 1 THEN
        ENTER PTDATA
      ENDIF
      IF PICK2 EQ 2 THEN
        ENTER PTSCHED
      ENDIF
      IF PICK2 EQ 3 THEN
        ENTER NEWADMIT
      ENDIF
      IF PICK2 EQ 4 THEN
        ENTER UNDER22
      ENDIF
      IF PICK2 EQ 5 THEN
        BREAK
      ENDIF
    ENDWHILE
    CLEAR LEVEL2
    CLEAR PICK2
```

```
      GOTO STARTAPP
 ENDIF
 IF PICK1 EQ 2 THEN
    SET VAR PICK2 INT
    SET VAR LEVEL2 INT
    SET VAR LEVEL2 TO 0
    WHILE LEVEL2 EQ 0 THEN
       NEWPAGE
       CHOOSE PICK2 FROM EDIT IN TICKLER.Apx
       IF PICK2 EQ 0 THEN
         BREAK
       ENDIF
       IF PICK2 EQ 1 THEN
         EDIT +
            ALL +
            FROM PTDATA +
            SORTED BY LNAME = A FRSTNAME = A
       ENDIF
       IF PICK2 EQ 2 THEN
         EDIT +
            ALL +
            FROM PTSCHED +
            SORTED BY CNO = A COMPDATE = A
         EDIT +
            ALL +
            FROM PTSCHED +
            SORTED BY CNO = A
       ENDIF
       IF PICK2 EQ 3 THEN
         EDIT +
            ALL +
            FROM NEWADMIT +
            SORTED BY CNO = A
       ENDIF
       IF PICK2 EQ 4 THEN
         EDIT +
            ALL +
            FROM UNDER22 +
            SORTED BY CNO = A
       ENDIF
       IF PICK2 EQ 5 THEN
```

```
            BREAK
          ENDIF
        ENDWHILE
        CLEAR LEVEL2
        CLEAR PICK2
        GOTO STARTAPP
    ENDIF
    IF PICK1 EQ 3 THEN
      SET VAR PICK2 INT
      SET VAR LEVEL2 INT
      SET VAR LEVEL2 TO 0
      WHILE LEVEL2 EQ 0 THEN
        NEWPAGE
        CHOOSE PICK2 FROM REPORTS IN TICKLER.Apx
        IF PICK2 EQ 1 THEN
          SET VAR PICK3 INT
          SET VAR LEVEL3 INT
          SET VAR LEVEL3 TO 0
          WHILE LEVEL3 EQ 0 THEN
            NEWPAGE
        CHOOSE PICK3 FROM REPORT1 IN TICKLER.Apx
        IF PICK3 EQ 0 THEN
            BREAK
        ENDIF
        IF PICK3 EQ 1 THEN
            CHOOSE PRNTOPT FROM PRT$$$ IN TICKLER.Apx
            IF PRNTOPT EQ "Both" THEN
              OUTPUT PRINTER WITH SCREEN
            ELSE
              IF PRNTOPT NE "Printer" THEN
                OUTPUT SCREEN
              ELSE
                OUTPUT PRINTER
              ENDIF
            ENDIF
            PRINT demog +
              SORTED BY WARD = A LNAME = A FRSTNAME = A
            OUTPUT SCREEN
            IF PRNTOPT NE "Printer" THEN
              WRITE "Press any key to continue"
              PAUSE
```

```
              ENDIF
              CLEAR PRNTOPT
          ENDIF
          IF PICK3 EQ 2 THEN
              CHOOSE PRNTOPT FROM PRT$$$ IN TICKLER.Apx
              IF PRNTOPT EQ "Both" THEN
                OUTPUT PRINTER WITH SCREEN
              ELSE
                IF PRNTOPT NE "Printer" THEN
                  OUTPUT SCREEN
                ELSE
                  OUTPUT PRINTER
                ENDIF
              ENDIF
              PRINT CLINICAL +
                SORTED BY WARD = A LNAME = A FRSTNAME = A
              OUTPUT SCREEN
              IF PRNTOPT NE "Printer" THEN
                WRITE "Press any key to continue"
                PAUSE
              ENDIF
              CLEAR PRNTOPT
          ENDIF
          IF PICK3 EQ 3 THEN
              CHOOSE PRNTOPT FROM PRT$$$ IN TICKLER.Apx
              IF PRNTOPT EQ "Both" THEN
                OUTPUT PRINTER WITH SCREEN
              ELSE
                IF PRNTOPT NE "Printer" THEN
                  OUTPUT SCREEN
              ELSE
                  OUTPUT PRINTER
                ENDIF
              ENDIF
              PRINT NEXTKIN +
                SORTED BY SW = A WARD = A LNAME = A
                FRSTNAME = A
              OUTPUT SCREEN
              IF PRNTOPT NE "Printer" THEN
                WRITE "Press any key to continue"
                PAUSE
```

```
    ENDIF
    CLEAR PRNTOPT
ENDIF
IF PICK3 EQ 4 THEN
    CHOOSE PRNTOPT FROM PRT$$$ IN TICKLER.Apx
    IF PRNTOPT EQ "Both" THEN
      OUTPUT PRINTER WITH SCREEN
    ELSE
      IF PRNTOPT NE "Printer" THEN
        OUTPUT SCREEN
      ELSE
        OUTPUT PRINTER
      ENDIF
    ENDIF
    PRINT TTL +
      SORTED BY TTL = A WARD = A LNAME = A
      FRSTNAME = A
    OUTPUT SCREEN
    IF PRNTOPT NE "Printer" THEN
      WRITE "Press any key to continue"
      PAUSE
    ENDIF
    CLEAR PRNTOPT
ENDIF
IF PICK3 EQ 5 THEN
ENDIF
IF PICK3 EQ 6 THEN
ENDIF
IF PICK3 EQ 7 THEN
    CHOOSE PRNTOPT FROM PRT$$$ IN TICKLER.Apx
    IF PRNTOPT EQ "Both" THEN
      OUTPUT PRINTER WITH SCREEN
    ELSE
      IF PRNTOPT NE "Printer" THEN
        OUTPUT SCREEN
      ELSE
        OUTPUT PRINTER
      ENDIF
    ENDIF
    PRINT UNDER22 +
      SORTED BY WARD = A LNAME = A FRSTNAME = A +
```

```
            WHERE AGE LE 22
            OUTPUT SCREEN
            IF PRNTOPT NE "Printer" THEN
              WRITE "Press any key to continue "
              PAUSE
            ENDIF
            CLEAR PRNTOPT
        ENDIF
        IF PICK3 EQ 8 THEN
            CHOOSE PRNTOPT FROM PRT$$$ IN TICKLER.Apx
            IF PRNTOPT EQ "Both" THEN
              OUTPUT PRINTER WITH SCREEN
            ELSE
              IF PRNTOPT NE "Printer" THEN
                OUTPUT SCREEN
              ELSE
                OUTPUT PRINTER
              ENDIF
            ENDIF
            PRINT NEWADMIT +
              SORTED BY WARD = A LNAME = A FRSTNAME = A +
              WHERE LOS LE 365
            OUTPUT SCREEN
            IF PRNTOPT NE "Printer" THEN
              WRITE "Press any key to continue"
              PAUSE
            ENDIF
            CLEAR PRNTOPT
        ENDIF
        IF PICK3 EQ 9 THEN
            BREAK
          ENDIF
        ENDWHILE
        CLEAR LEVEL3
        CLEAR PICK3
    ENDIF
    IF PICK2 EQ 2 THEN
        SET VAR PICK3 INT
        SET VAR LEVEL3 INT
        SET VAR LEVEL3 TO 0
        WHILE LEVEL3 EQ 0 THEN
```

```
NEWPAGE
CHOOSE PICK3 FROM REPORT2 IN TICKLER.Apx
IF PICK3 EQ 0 THEN
    BREAK
ENDIF
IF PICK3 EQ 1 THEN
    CHOOSE PRNTOPT FROM PRT$$$ IN TICKLER.Apx
    IF PRNTOPT EQ "Both" THEN
      OUTPUT PRINTER WITH SCREEN
    ELSE
      IF PRNTOPT NE "Printer" THEN
        OUTPUT SCREEN
      ELSE
        OUTPUT PRINTER
      ENDIF
    ENDIF
    PRINT ACTRPRT +
        SORTED BY WARD = A ACTIVDUE = A +
        WHERE ACTIVDUE LE      .#DATE
    OUTPUT SCREEN
    IF PRNTOPT NE "Printer" THEN
        WRITE "Press any key to continue"
        PAUSE
    ENDIF
    CLEAR PRNTOPT
ENDIF
IF PICK3 EQ 2 THEN
    CHOOSE PRNTOPT FROM PRT$$$ IN TICKLER.Apx
    IF PRNTOPT EQ "Both" THEN
        OUTPUT PRINTER WITH SCREEN
    ELSE
        IF PRNTOPT NE "Printer" THEN
          OUTPUT SCREEN
        ELSE
          OUTPUT PRINTER
        ENDIF
    ENDIF
    PRINT COMPRPRT +
        SORTED BY WARD = A COMPDUE = A +
        WHERE COMPDUE LE      .#DATE
    OUTPUT SCREEN
```

```
IF PRNTOPT NE "Printer" THEN
    WRITE "Press any key to continue"
    PAUSE
ENDIF
CLEAR PRNTOPT
ENDIF
IF PICK3 EQ 3 THEN
CHOOSE PRNTOPT FROM PRT$$$ IN TICKLER.Apx
IF PRNTOPT EQ "Both" THEN
    OUTPUT PRINTER WITH SCREEN
ELSE
    IF PRNTOPT NE "Printer" THEN
        OUTPUT SCREEN
    ELSE
        OUTPUT PRINTER
    ENDIF
ENDIF
PRINT ASSESSMT +
    SORTED BY WARD = A LNAME = A FRSTNAME = A
OUTPUT SCREEN
IF PRNTOPT NE "Printer" THEN
    WRITE "Press any key to continue"
    PAUSE
ENDIF
CLEAR PRNTOPT ENDIF
IF PICK3 EQ 4 THEN
CHOOSE PRNTOPT FROM PRT$$$ IN TICKLER.Apx
IF PRNTOPT EQ "Both" THEN
    OUTPUT PRINTER WITH SCREEN
ELSE
    IF PRNTOPT NE "Printer" THEN
        OUTPUT SCREEN
    ELSE
        OUTPUT PRINTER
    ENDIF
ENDIF
PRINT EDRPRT +
    SORTED BY EDUCDUE = A
OUTPUT SCREEN
IF PRNTOPT NE "Printer" THEN
    WRITE "Press any key to continue"
```

```
        PAUSE
ENDIF
CLEAR PRNTOPT
CHOOSE PRNTOPT FROM PRT$$$ IN TICKLER.Apx
IF PRNTOPT EQ "Both" THEN
        OUTPUT PRINTER WITH SCREEN
ELSE
        IF PRNTOPT NE "Printer" THEN
          OUTPUT SCREEN
        ELSE
          OUTPUT PRINTER
        ENDIF
ENDIF
PRINT EDRPRT +
        SORTED BY WARD = A EDUCDUE = A +
        WHERE EDUCDUE LE      .#DATE
OUTPUT SCREEN
IF PRNTOPT NE "Printer" THEN
        WRITE "Press any key to continue"
        PAUSE
        ENDIF
        CLEAR PRNTOPT
ENDIF
IF PICK3 EQ 5 THEN
        CHOOSE PRNTOPT FROM PRT$$$ IN TICKLER.Apx
        IF PRNTOPT EQ "Both" THEN
          OUTPUT PRINTER WITH SCREEN
        ELSE
          IF PRNTOPT NE "Printer" THEN
            OUTPUT SCREEN
          ELSE
            OUTPUT PRINTER
        ENDIF
ENDIF
PRINT NURSRPRT +
        SORTED BY WARD = A NURSDUE = A +
        WHERE NURSDUE LE      .#DATE
OUTPUT SCREEN
IF PRNTOPT NE "Printer" THEN
        WRITE "Press any key to continue"
        PAUSE
```

```
        ENDIF
        CLEAR PRNTOPT
     ENDIF
     IF PICK3 EQ 6 THEN
        CHOOSE PRNTOPT FROM PRT$$$ IN TICKLER.Apx
        IF PRNTOPT EQ "Both" THEN
            OUTPUT PRINTER WITH SCREEN
        ELSE
            IF PRNTOPT NE "Printer" THEN
               OUTPUT SCREEN
            ELSE
               OUTPUT PRINTER
            ENDIF
        ENDIF
        PRINT NUTRPRT +
            SORTED BY WARD = A NUTDUE = A +
            WHERE NUTDUE LE     .#DATE
        OUTPUT SCREEN
        IF PRNTOPT NE "Printer" THEN
            WRITE "Press any key to continue"
            PAUSE
        ENDIF
        CLEAR PRNTOPT
     ENDIF
     IF PICK3 EQ 7 THEN
        CHOOSE PRNTOPT FROM PRT$$$ IN TICKLER.Apx
        IF PRNTOPT EQ "Both" THEN
            OUTPUT PRINTER WITH SCREEN
        ELSE
            IF PRNTOPT NE "Printer" THEN
               OUTPUT SCREEN
            ELSE
               OUTPUT PRINTER
            ENDIF
        ENDIF
        PRINT PSOLRPRT +
            SORTED BY WARD = A PSOLDUE = A +
            WHERE PSOLDUE LE     .#DATE
        OUTPUT SCREEN
        IF PRNTOPT NE "Printer" THEN
            WRITE "Press any key to continue"
```

```
            PAUSE
        ENDIF
        CLEAR PRNTOPT
    ENDIF
    IF PICK3 EQ 8 THEN
            CHOOSE PRNTOPT FROM PRT$$$ IN TICKLER.Apx
            IF PRNTOPT EQ "Both" THEN
              OUTPUT PRINTER WITH SCREEN
            ELSE
              IF PRNTOPT NE "Printer" THEN
                OUTPUT SCREEN
              ELSE
                OUTPUT PRINTER
              ENDIF
            ENDIF
            PRINT PSYRPRT +
              SORTED BY WARD = A PSYCHDUE = A +
              WHERE PSYCHDUE LE      .#DATE
            OUTPUT SCREEN
            IF PRNTOPT NE "Printer" THEN
              WRITE "Press any key to continue"
              PAUSE
            ENDIF
            CLEAR PRNTOPT
        ENDIF
        IF PICK3 EQ 9 THEN
            BREAK
        ENDIF
    ENDWHILE
    CLEAR LEVEL3
    CLEAR PICK3
ENDIF
IF PICK2 EQ 3 THEN
    SET VAR PICK3 INT
    SET VAR LEVEL3 INT
    SET VAR LEVEL3 TO 0
    WHILE LEVEL3 EQ 0 THEN
      NEWPAGE
      CHOOSE PICK3 FROM REPORT3 IN TICKLER.Apx
      IF PICK3 EQ 0 THEN
          BREAK
```

```
ENDIF
IF PICK3 EQ 1 THEN
    CHOOSE PRNTOPT FROM PRT$$$ IN TICKLER.Apx
    IF PRNTOPT EQ "Both" THEN
      OUTPUT PRINTER WITH SCREEN
    ELSE
      IF PRNTOPT NE "Printer" THEN
        OUTPUT SCREEN
    ELSE
        OUTPUT PRINTER
    ENDIF
ENDIF
PRINT PXRPRT +
    SORTED BY WARD = A PXDUE = A +
    WHERE PXDUE LE      .#DATE
OUTPUT SCREEN
IF PRNTOPT NE "Printer" THEN
    WRITE "Press any key to continue"
    PAUSE
ENDIF
CLEAR PRNTOPT
ENDIF
IF PICK3 EQ 2 THEN
  CHOOSE PRNTOPT FROM PRT$$$ IN TICKLER.Apx
  IF PRNTOPT EQ "Both" THEN
      OUTPUT PRINTER WITH SCREEN
  ELSE
      IF PRNTOPT NE "Printer" THEN
        OUTPUT SCREEN
      ELSE
        OUTPUT PRINTER
      ENDIF
  ENDIF
  PRINT SOCREPRT +
      SORTED BY WARD = A SOCDUE = A +
      WHERE SOCDUE LE      .#DATE
  OUTPUT SCREEN
  IF PRNTOPT NE "Printer" THEN
      WRITE "Press any key to continue"
      PAUSE
  ENDIF
```

```
    CLEAR PRNTOPT
ENDIF
IF PICK3 EQ 3 THEN
    CHOOSE PRNTOPT FROM PRT$$$ IN TICKLER.Apx
    IF PRNTOPT EQ "Both" THEN
        OUTPUT PRINTER WITH SCREEN
    ELSE
        IF PRNTOPT NE "Printer" THEN
          OUTPUT SCREEN
        ELSE
        OUTPUT PRINTER
        ENDIF
    ENDIF
    PRINT VOCRPRT +
        SORTED BY WARD = A VOCDUE = A +
        WHERE VOCDUE LE      .#DATE
    OUTPUT SCREEN
    IF PRNTOPT NE "Printer" THEN
        WRITE "Press any key to continue"
        PAUSE
    ENDIF
    CLEAR PRNTOPT
ENDIF
IF PICK3 EQ 4 THEN
    CHOOSE PRNTOPT FROM PRT$$$ IN TICKLER.Apx
    IF PRNTOPT EQ "Both" THEN
        OUTPUT PRINTER WITH SCREEN
    ELSE
        IF PRNTOPT NE "Printer" THEN
          OUTPUT SCREEN
        ELSE
          OUTPUT PRINTER
        ENDIF
    ENDIF
    PRINT QUARPRT +
        SORTED BY WARD = A QUARTDUE = A +
        WHERE QUARTDUE LE      .#DATE
    OUTPUT SCREEN
    IF PRNTOPT NE "Printer" THEN
        WRITE "Press any key to continue"
        PAUSE
```

```
      ENDIF
      CLEAR PRNTOPT
    ENDIF
    IF PICK3 EQ 5 THEN
      BREAK
      ENDIF
    ENDWHILE
    CLEAR LEVEL3
    CLEAR PICK3
    ENDIF
    IF PICK2 EQ 4 THEN
        BREAK
      ENDIF
    ENDWHILE
    CLEAR LEVEL2
    CLEAR PICK2
    GOTO STARTAPP
ENDIF
IF PICK1 EQ 4 THEN
  SET VAR PICK2 INT
  SET VAR LEVEL2 INT
  SET VAR LEVEL2 TO 0
  WHILE LEVEL2 EQ 0 THEN
      NEWPAGE
      CHOOSE PICK2 FROM DELETE IN TICKLER.Apx
      IF PICK2 EQ 0 THEN
        BREAK
      ENDIF
      IF PICK2 EQ 1 THEN
        SET VARIABLE WHVAL1        TEXT
        FILLIN WHVAL1 USING "ENTER PATIENT "CNO"TO
BE DELETED"
        DELETE ROWS FROM PTDATA +
          WHERE CNO      EQ.        WHVAL1
        CLEAR WHVAL1
      ENDIF
      IF PICK2 EQ 2 THEN
        SET VARIABLE WHVAL1 TEXT
        FILLIN WHVAL1 USING "ENTER PATIENT CNO TO
        BE DELETED"
        DELETE ROWS FROM PTSCHED +
```

```
          WHERE CNO      EQ.        WHVAL1
          CLEAR WHVAL1
     ENDIF
     IF PICK2 EQ 3 THEN
        SET VARIABLE WHVAL1 TEXT
        FILLIN WHVAL1 USING "ENTER PATIENT CNO TO
        BE DELETED"
          DELETE ROWS FROM NEWADMIT +
            WHERE CNO      EQ.        WHVAL1
          CLEAR WHVAL1
        ENDIF
        IF PICK2 EQ 4 THEN
          SET VARIABLE WHVAL1 TEXT
          FILLIN WHVAL1 USING "ENTER PATIENT CNO TO
          BE DELETED"
          DELETE ROWS FROM UNDER22 +
            WHERE CNO      EQ.        WHVAL1
          CLEAR WHVAL1
        ENDIF
        IF PICK2 EQ 5 THEN
          BREAK
        ENDIF
      ENDWHILE
      CLEAR LEVEL2
      CLEAR PICK2
      GOTO STARTAPP
      ENDIF
      IF PICK1 EQ 5 THEN
        GOTO ENDAPP
      ENDIF
      GOTO STARTAPP
LABEL ENDAPP
CLEAR PICK1
RETURN
$MENU
PRT$$$
ROW Select Print Routing
Printer
Screen
Both
$MENU
```

Main
COLUMN TICKLER SYSTEM MAIN MENU
ENTER DATA
EDIT DATA
PRINT REPORTS
DELETE DATA
EXIT$MENU
INPUT
COLUMN DATA ENTRY MENU
PATIENT BASIC DATA
ASSESSMENT DATES
PERIODIC REVIEW—NEWLY ADMITTED
PERIODIC REVIEW—UNDER AGE 22
RETURN TO MAIN MENU
$MENU
REPORTS
COLUMN PRINTED REPORTS MENU
PATIENT CHARACTERISTICS REPORT
ASSESSMENTS DUE DATES REPORTS
MORE ASSESSMENT DUE DATES REPORTS
EXIT TO TICKLER
$MENU
REPORT1
COLUMN PATIENTS CHARACTERISTICS REPORTS
PATIENT DEMOGRAPHIC PROFILE BY WARD
PATIENT CLINICAL INFORMATION BY WARD
PATIENT NEXT OF KIN REPORT BY SOCIAL WOKER
LISTING OF PATIENTS BY TEAM LEADERS
LISTING OF PATIENTS BY PHYSICIAN
LISTING OF PATIENTS BY LENGTH OF STAY
PERIODIC REVIEW SCHEDULE—PATIENT UNDER AGE 22
PERIODIC REVIEW SCHEDULE—PATIENT NEWLY ADMITTED
RETURN TO REPORT MENU
$MENU
REPORT2
COLUMN ASSESSMENTS DUE DATES REPORTS—CHOOSE A RE-
PORT
ACTIVITY ASSESSMENTS
COMPREHENSIVE ASSESSMENT
LISTING OF ALL ASSESSMENTS DUE DATES BY WARD
EDUCATIONAL ASSESSMENT

NURSING ASSESSMENT
NUTRITION ASSESSMENT
PSYCHOLOGICAL ASSESSMENT
PSYCHIATRIC ASSESSMENT
RETURN TO REPORTS MENU FOR MORE ASSESSMENT RE-
PORTS
$MENU
REPORT3
COLUMN MORE ASSESSMENT REPORTS
PHYSICAL EXAMINATION REPORT
SOCIAL ASSESSMENT REPORT
VOCATIONAL ASSESSMENT REPORT
QUARTERLY REVIEW DATES
EXIT TO REPORT MENU
$MENU
DELETE
COLUMN DELETE DATA MENU
PATIENT BASIC DATA
ASSESSMENTS DATA
NEWLY ADMITTED PATIENT
PATIENT UNDER AGE 22
EXIT$MENU
EDIT
COLUMN EDIT DATA MENU
EDIT PATIENT BASIC DATA
EDIT PATIENT ASSESSMENT DUE DATES
EDIT PERIODIC REVIEW DATES – NEWLY ADMITTED PATIENTS
EDIT PERIODIC REVIEW DATES – PATIENTS UNDER AGE 22
EXIT

Speech Timing
of Mood Disorders

Ernest H. Friedman
Gary G. Sanders

KEYWORDS. Computerized evaluation of speech, speech pauses, coronary risks, mood disorders, schizophrenia

SUMMARY. Computerized evaluation of pauses between spoken words can be conducted in the medical office or over the telephone. Frequency and duration of long speech hesitation pauses (LP = > 1 sec.) can be correlated with coronary-risk and mood. Pauses of 100 + msec are sorted into many fluency levels. Peak fluency of LP irrespective of pause-time, and at maximal pause-time, are behavioral correlates of mood. At intermediate fluency they are explained by left-hemisphere, right-hemisphere and interhemispheric transit, respectively. Short pauses (SP = < 1 sec.) sorted at these fluency nodes monitor competence of asymmetric and interhemispheric brain functions. Diurnal mood variation is monitored by comparing the morning and evening frequency and duration of the patient's pauses. The frequency of pauses within < 1.16 second may diagnose manic mood modulated by the basal region of the right temporal lobe. LP and SP may monitor interrelationships among mood and thought disorders subserved by the left dorsal prefrontal cortex.

BACKGROUND

Speech, which may be defined as the faculty or ability to convey thoughts or ideas by the generation of intelligible acoustic patterns, is not unique to humans if one considers the mating, alarm, flock-

Ernest H. Friedman, MD, is a practicing psychiatrist with an interest in the psychosocial factors of coronary risk. He is a member of the Departments of Medicine and Psychiatry at: Case Western Reserve University, 1831 Forest Hills Boulevard, East Cleveland, OH 44112-4313. Gary G. Sanders, BSEE, MT, FICMT, is a design engineer in medical technology at Penberthy Inc., 3104 Prophetstown Rd., Rock Falls, IL 61071.

121

ing, etc., sounds made by various animal species. Unique to humans within the animal kingdom is the high degree of complexity, structuralization and systemization of sounds codified into languages. This allows the conveyance of complex ideas among species members. This ability has a cost which is the amount of brain resource utilization employed. Consider what is required, using concept transfer as the model. First the brain must conjure up the abstract premise and form it into a logical flow. From this point the idea must be associated with sound patterns (words) that are part of the resident vocabulary. This outline function must then be polished with the addition of the grammatical structures appropriate to the language. Then the complex interaction of multiple muscular systems (from the diaphragm up through the nasal cavities) must be coordinated to achieve the desired sound pattern generation as well as facial expressions and 'body language' that accompany speech and all within short time frames, as compared with writing where the complexity may be similar but the time frame is extended.

Reflection will reveal that no other single human endeavor besides speech places such a demanding load on the available brain resources. This load can in turn affect cardiac function. The relationship is illustrated by a causal link shown between a personally relevant speaking task and myocardial ischemia of a similar magnitude as exercise. It is also illustrated by speech hesitation pauses > 1 second in length > 2 times per minute that predicted sixfold higher coronary incidence in 2 groups of otherwise normal coronary-prone men followed prospectively for 10 years (Friedman & Sanders, 1988).

Measurement of pauses in speech has a history going back 3,000 years. In India, pauses were called "kali," which included short pauses for breathing and long pauses for meaning (Savithri, 1988). Alcibiades, the ancient Greek orator, often hesitated in the midst of a speech causing audiences to hang on his words (Safire, 1991). In the thirteenth century, medieval musicians added pauses in the development of polyphonic music which until that time lacked rests. Philosophers of that day were mainly influenced by Aristotle's idea that time was related primarily to motion. One author (probably a Parisian student) wrote a chapter on pauses in "The Notre Dame Notations" and used the pseudonym "Anonymous IV" to avoid an accusation of heresy (Szamosi, 1986).

In the eighteenth century, Jonathan Steele in England wrote a book titled "PROSODIA RATIONALIS" demonstrating the role of pauses in rhythmic expressions and used this to analyze the works of Shakespeare (Steele, 1779). In the 1960's in England, Basil Bernstein (1962) described longer pauses for effective planning and Frieda Goldman-Eisler's psycholinguistic studies showed variations in pauses for emphasis (1968).

In 1963, Joseph Jaffe defined a set of vocal parameters that would be concerned only with verbal behavior (i.e., would not include gestures and would not be inferred from the content of a monologue or dialogue) and which could be automatically obtained from live or audiotaped dialogues (Jaffe & Feldstein, 1970).

MECHANICAL EVALUATION OF PAUSES

Cassotta described an analogue-to-digital analysis system in 1964 called the Automatic Vocal Transaction Analyzer (AVTA) (Welkowitz et al., 1990). The analog voltage signal of each speaker's channel triggered a voice relay that sampled the presence or absence of sounds at a fixed sampling rate. Investigators using this system and its later modifications have primarily been concerned with examination of the frequencies and durations of turns, vocalizations, hesitation pauses, switching pauses, and simultaneous speech (interruptions). A turn is an interval beginning the instant one participant in a conversation starts to talk alone and ends immediately prior to the instant another participant starts to talk alone. It is thus defined as the time during which a participant has the floor and indexes the feature that defines a conversation, that is, the fact that its participants alternate or take turns speaking. Other vocal parameters represent events that occur within each participant's turn. A vocalization is a continuous, uninterrupted segment of speech (sound) uttered by the person who has the floor. The switching pause is an interval of joint silence bounded by the vocalizations of different participants, that is, it follows a vocalization of another participant who thereby obtains the floor. Thus, it is a silence that marks a switch of speakers. Hesitation pauses during dialogues are defined as joint silences bounded by the speech of one of the conversational partners. Simultaneous speech is speech uttered by a participant who does not have the floor during a vocalization by the participant who does have the floor. On the basis of its outcome, simultaneous speech may be divided into two types, interruptive and noninterruptive. Noninterruptive simultaneous speech begins and ends while the participant who has the floor is talking. Interruptive simultaneous speech is part of a speech segment that begins while the person who has the floor is talking and ends after he/she has stopped.

Martz and Welkowitz (1977) developed programs (dubbed WELMAR) to analyze sequences of sounds and silences, i.e., turns, vocalizations, hesitation pauses, switching pauses, and simultaneous speech, using small computers. A two-channel recorder and two level meters were connected to two analog-to-digital converter channels of a PDP-12 computer. A computer program transformed the analog wave shapes from the sound level meters that represented the two speakers' vocal intensities into two interleaved digital series and stored these data on LINC tapes. A series of software programs were written to analyze the frequencies and durations of the vocal parameters. A major addition in WELMAR II is a time series regression program that provides a way of examining directional influence in two-person interactions. The use of computers thus shows great promise in helping researchers understand basic properties of the communication process (Welkowitz et al., 1990).

Responsive understanding with delayed action (Bakhtin, 1986) and the correlation of the frequency and duration of hesitation pauses to coronary-risk and mood, respectively, confirmed the need to detect longer but less recurrent pauses (i.e., echo-time in the right hemisphere for reflection) (Friedman & Sanders, 1988).

VOXAFLEX SPEECH ANALYSIS

Speech pause time is acquired by external hardware coupled to a PC type microcomputer. The external hardware has one PVDF acoustic transducer with a cardioid (limacon of Pascal with a = b) pattern integral for use in monologue acquisition or as the local voice transducer for dialogues. For dialogues another acoustic transducer, either fitted to a telephone's handset receiver (allowing remote acquisition) or with other forms of restricted pattern is added. The external hardware has two channels each with cascade 12dB/octave rolloff bandpass ($f_l = 300$ Hz, $f_h = 3$ KHz) amplifiers (total A_v adjustable 8 to 114 dB-normal gain setting is 55 dB) followed by a saturating amplifier. These stages output a digitally compatible pulse train. This pulse train is processed through an F-to-V converter into a window comparator setup as a 'brick wall' (i.e., infinite slope skirt) bandpass filter ($f_l = 330$ Hz, $f_h = 2.7$ KHz). The outputs of the two channels are then logically combined and analyzed further.

Telephone acquisition of speech pauses follows a different method. It uses differential gain between the side-tones generated locally at the receiver compared with the local acoustic transducer in contrast to the remotely generated voice. Switching of the logic and power for the telephone transducer is accomplished when the transducer is plugged into the unit. The decoded outputs are electrically converted to RS232C standards and brought out to a DB-9 connector. This is wired to a serial (COM) port on a PC type microcomputer which when running the acquisition (monitoring) software, provides all of the timing and translation necessary to store the acquired data as a compressed file. Information tagged into the file includes participant's name(s), timing information, calendar date, time, and other housekeeping information.

File name generation is automatic and forms the basis of a mini indexed database system that provides for sorting and recalling the files on several search criteria. The filed data have only timing information, with no verbiage storage, thus ensuring privacy of communication. The analysis portion of the software post-processes either newly acquired or recalled data. Post-processing is predicated upon a mixture of defined brain timing (as verified by EEG, MRI, PET, etc.) and statistical derivatives. The output of the program is a variety of screen displays. A print option exists which is a replica of the active display with additional information.

EVALUATION OF SPEECH DATA

Speech hesitation pauses of 100 or more milliseconds are analyzed on a time-base and sorted into various fluency levels. Peak fluency of long pauses (LP: defined as $> = 1$ second) irrespective of pause-time, at maximal pause-time, a behavioral correlate of mood, and at intermediate fluencies are left-hemisphere node (LH), right-hemisphere node (RH), and interhemispheric transit nodes (LT: left interhemispheric transit / CT: callosal transit / RT: right interhemispheric transit), respectively. These fluency nodes approximate when asymmetric and interhemispheric brain functions are synchronized for complex tasks, expressed as a SYNCHRONY INDEX. Productivity of the hemispheres is compared by speech time/floor time (speech time + pause-time) at LH vs RH nodes expressed as a BALANCE INDEX. Short pauses (SP: defined as less than 1 second) sorted at these fluency nodes monitor competence of asymmetric and interhemispheric brain functions expressed as COMPETENCE INDEXES in tabular and graphic form accompanied by manic < 1 δ LP time [+], depressed > 1 δ LP time [-], and very depressed > 2 δ LP time [−] moods. Participatory matching indicated by a COMM INDEX monitors a joint mutually responsive rhythm (Friedman, 1989a; Friedman, 1989b; Friedman 1990a). The neural substrate is suggested by delay-dependent speeding of reaction time reflecting motor readiness abolished by depletion of dopamine (Brown & Robbins, 1991).

CLINICAL APPLICATIONS OF SPEECH ANALYSIS

The need for improved recognition and treatment of mood disorders is evidenced from surveys of patients defined as refractory in tertiary care settings. A majority including a group referred for psychosurgery, had simply not received adequately intensive psychopharmacological treatment. Consistent with the evidence for the under-treatment of depression, manic-depressive-illness is both under-recognized and under-treated (Guscott & Grof, 1991). Goodwin and Jamison (1990) estimated that no more than one-third of patients with manic-depressive illness receive treatment. This claim is supported by the study of Schou and Weeke (1988), who described the undertreatment of patients with affective disorders who committed suicide. They concluded that many of these patients could have benefitted from either continuation or prophylactic treatment with antidepressants or lithium. The findings from tertiary care settings are consistent with the research on the diagnosis and treatment of depression in primary care. The undertreatment of depression is still a major problem (Guscott & Grof, 1991).

Precise diagnosis and response to treatment of mood disorders can be facilitated by analyzing speech pauses on a time-base (Friedman & Sanders, 1988). Diagnosis of bipolar "rate" disorder (Hyde, 1990) by monitoring speech pause-time, 1.50 $+/-$ 0.33 sec. (Mean $+/-$ δ), a behavioral correlate of mood (Friedman & Sanders, 1988) is suggested by a dopamine-dependent internal clock (Rammsayer, 1990), by lateralization of pause-time and dopamine to the right hemisphere (Friedman & Benson, 1990; Gambert et al., 1991), and by dopamine depletion abolishing delay-dependent speeded reaction time indicative of motor readiness (Brown & Robbins, 1991). It also is suggested by a major role for the basal region of the right temporal lobe in the modulation of mood (Friedman & Robinson, 1991), by a significant negative correlation between the duration of illness and right temporal lobe volume in men with refractory bipolar disorder (Altshuler et al., 1991), and by long-term rapid cycling unchanged by bifrontal lobectomy in an 81-year-old woman (Mizukawa et al., 1991) whose right hemisphere was at a higher metabolic rate (Gambert et al., 1991). The role of the right hemisphere is supported by slower reaction times to the left visual field (right hemisphere) in mild unipolar depression (Liotti et al., 1991).

The "switch process" and rapid cycling in manic-depressive illness (Bunney & Hartmann, 1965; Bunney et al., 1972a; Bunney et al., 1972b; Bunney et al., 1972c; Mizukawa et al., 1991) may be monitored by the neural basis of the detection by a receiver (Friedman, 1990a) of the temporal features of expressive activity analyzing speech pauses on a time-base, reflecting internal state (Halliday & Houston, 1991), whose validity is a function of reproducibility across time, circumstance, diagnosis, race, and specie (Friedman, 1991a; Pindzola, 1990). Pause measurement can develop a differential typology that examines competence, efficiency and speed of asymmetric and interhemispheric brain functions (Friedman & Sanders, 1988; Friedman, 1989a; Friedman, 1990a; Welford, 1988) to reach beyond the results that can be achieved by means of a static psychopathological morphology, especially considering the improved prognostic validity of psychiatric diagnoses (Braunig, 1990). This method may shed light on the causes of biological rhythm change during manic-depressive illness with aging manifested by prolongation of affective days in both manic and depressive episodes. Longitudinal monitoring demonstrated 64 switches into mania in 10 years in an 81-year-old woman, 52 of which (81.3%) occurred between 11 PM and 8 AM. Furthermore, 28 of the 52 switches happened between 2 am and 6 am. Lying in bed all day in the depressive phase (Mizukawa et al., 1991) suggests temperamental differences in gender-mediated clinical features of depressive illness manifested by women's less active, more ruminative responses linked to dysfunction in the right frontal cortex (Friedman & Jacobs, 1991).

Gender-related cerebral asymmetries manifested by dysregulation of right frontal lobe function (Friedman & Jacobs, 1991) during manic episodes by abnormalities of the basal region of the right temporal lobe (Friedman, 1990c; Friedman & Robinson, 1991) are suggested by diminished antitrichotillomanic effects of clomipramine in four women which may have been due to extended periods of affective stimulation (Pollard et al., 1991), and by successful lithium treatment of hair pulling predominantly in women (9 of 10) (Christenson et al., 1991). They also are suggested by neurophysiologic dysfunction in basal ganglia/limbic striatal and thalamocortical circuits considered to be a pathogenetic mechanism of obsessive-compulsive disorder (OCD) (Modell et al., 1989), by basal ganglia and/or right hemisphere disturbance documented in OCD patients in positron emission tomography and magnetic resonance imaging investigations (Boone et al., 1991), and by nonverbal, perhaps nondominant hemisphere or subcortical processing deficits in OCD patients (Zielinski et al., 1991).

Microcomputer based data acquisition of speech pauses may be conducted by telephone to monitor diurnal mood variation not easily apparent during single, isolated interviews. Percent of elapsed times of patient-therapist dialogues more than 1.83 sec. or less than 1.17 sec. indicate depression and mania respectively (Friedman &

Robinson, 1991). This strategy is supported by participatory matching that has prelinguistic origins ensuring a joint, mutually responsive rhythm (Friedman, 1989b) mediated by the right hemisphere (Fries & Swihart, 1990; O'Boyle et al., 1990), and by rhythmic activity in the neocortex generated or promoted by layer 5 pyramidal neurons manifested by epochs 1 to 4 sec in duration recurring spontaneously one to nine times/min. (Silva et al., 1991). It also is supported by long pauses (LP:1 + sec.), > 2 per minute, 4.79 +/ − 2.48 per min. subserved by Broca's area in the left hemisphere, predicting 6:1 coronary incidence in 2 groups of normal coronary-prone men followed prospectively for 10 years, p < .05 (Friedman & Sanders, 1988), by a causal link between a personally relevant speaking task and myocardial ischemia of a similar magnitude as exercise (Friedman, 1990b), and by a stress-activated neural link that may be involved in the pathogenetic process of coronary vasospasm (Natelson et al., 1991). These findings are supported by non-invasive rapid transcranial magnetic stimulation over the left hemisphere inducing speech arrest leading to bursts of crying (Pascual-Leone et al., 1991), and by inactivation of the left hemisphere manifested by increased speech hesitation, heart rate and emotionality (Friedman, 1991c; Friedman, 1991d; Stagno et al., 1990).

The absence of pauses during counting errors induced at lower intensity, tends to support the role of cognitive tasks in the systematic study of biphemispheric cortical organization of language (Pascual-Leone et al., 1991). This method may be applied to patients with coronary heart disease and altered temporal patterns of work to establish whether the end points of coronary disease are related primarily to the sleep-wake period or to identifiable periods of increased activity or stress during daily life (Mulcahy et al., 1991). Silent intervals in communication are demonstrated by courtship responses of female canaries after lesions of a forebrain nucleus resulting in failure to discriminate between male roller canary song lasting 5.4 +/− 3.0 sec. separated by silent intervals of 1.8 +/− 0.9 sec., and white-crowned sparrow song lasting 1.55 sec. repeated at intervals of 2.45 sec. (Brenowitz, 1991), by anticipatory synchrony of chirps every 2.1 sec. by Mecopoda S (Friedman,

1991a), and by perception of speech rate from the sound-silence patterns of monologues (Crown & Feldstein, 1991) mediated by the left cerebral hemisphere (Robin et al., 1990).

The inverse correlation of the frequency and duration of pauses to talking speed (Crystal & House, 1982), the higher quality, less interruptive Type A structured interviews manifested by longer turn-taking pauses in the Western Collaborative Group Study, 1.82 +/ − 0.63 sec. compared with the Multiple Risk Factor Intervention Trial, 1.00 +/− 0.38 sec., p <.01 (Tallmer et al., 1990), and a high emphasis/moderate warmth interview style with pausing slightly after the enunciation of key words resulting in a greater degree of engagement of the interviewee (Fontana et al., 1990) tend to support the greater accuracy of pauses compared with decreased vocal inflection in the measurement of dysprosody in Broca's aphasia (Friedman & Benson, 1990). Participatory matching, at 2 pauses per min., which is optimal performance at moderate arousal, is a joint, mutually responsive rhythm (Friedman, 1989b) that addresses the growing body of evidence concerning associations between differential interactional histories and attachment quality (Isabella & Belsky, 1991). Motor patterns are overproduced during a particular phase of ontogeny, and are then subjected to attrition and selective reinforcement by various kinds of social stimulation as maturation occurs (Marler, 1991). Amodal brain-based language acquisition is demonstrated by gestural babbling in deaf infants (Petitto & Marentette, 1991). The ability to modify vocal sounds by reference to auditory feedback, and blurring of the demarcation between what is an auditory and what is a motor circuit, call for a reassessment of the mechanisms and origins of vocal learning in birds and mammals (Nottebohm, 1991).

Speech timing can be applied to coronary-prone behavior monitored by pauses plotted on a time-base that can be integrated with antemortem markers and population and molecular genetic studies. It can also identify cerebral asymmetries in early Alzheimer's disease and increased susceptibility to dementia based on an underlying biological predisposition, and to monitor the rate of disease progression manifested by diminishing brain reserve.

Gender-related cerebral asymmetries are suggested by women with myocardial infarction exhibiting a fivefold higher prevalence rate of Alzheimer's disease linked to dopamine abnormalities and inefficient cortical circuits in the right-hemisphere (Gambert et al., 1991). These findings are supported by a fivefold higher prevalence rate of dementia in blacks, peaking in women, possibly related to a history of stroke and hypertension (Heyman et al., 1991). The trend is also supported by right frontal dysfunction in females (Friedman & Jacobs, 1991).

Dopaminergic stimulation may reduce cognitive processing speed (Poewe et al., 1991), and excessive L-dopa, an intermediate in the biosynthesis of dopamine, may cause neurodegeneration (Taylor, 1991).

Speech pause time, a behavioral correlate of mood, is a precise indicator of adequate antidepressant treatment for the reversible dementia of depression ("pseudodementia"), as distinguished from early Alzheimer's disease. Pauses processed on a time-base and sorted into many fluency levels may monitor coping skills, adjustment to the environment, neural substrates, the effect of medication, and provide more accurate guidelines than have previously been available for activities where performance impairment is a factor, such as independent living and driving an automobile (Gambert et al., 1991; Gilley et al., 1991; Kruger, 1989). The need to monitor gender-related cerebral asymmetries prospectively, is supported by inefficient cortical circuits in the right-hemisphere which may increase vulnerability to akathisia in women due to iron-dependent dopamine-D2 receptor hypofunction (Barton et al., 1990; Brown et al., 1987; Nemes et al., 1991). It also is supported by gaze and thought disorders in women linked to right frontal cortex dysfunction (Gambert et al., 1991; Friedman & Jacobs, 1991) that may include blindness with intact vision in Cambodian women correlated with the amount of time spent under horrible conditions (Cooke, 1991). Regional neurotransmitter imbalance (Gambert et al., 1991) may be manifested by delay-dependent speeding of reaction time abolished by depletion of dopamine indicated by LP 1.50 sec. accompanied by elongated switching pauses < 1 sec. (Brown & Robbins, 1991).

Diurnal mood variation in depression following stroke and reverse diurnal variation in panic disorder (Friedman & Robinson, 1991; Friedman, 1991e) support the sensitivity of pauses to dimensions of personality and psychological pathology (Welkowitz et al., 1990). The role of temporal processing in dyslexia, evaluated by an interstimulus interval of 2 sec. and 3 sec. display duration providing ample time to identify all words, is supported by the coexistence of attention deficit disorder and depression monitored by speech pause time, 1.50 +/− 0.33 sec. (Friedman, 1991a).

CLINICAL CASE EXAMPLES

A schizophrenic patient with drug related side effects was monitored by speech pause technology:

> A 39-year-old paranoid schizophrenic female (G.B.) gave a history of auditory hallucinations during an oculogyric crisis when treated with haloperidol 5 mg TID in July, 1990, in another city one month before returning to Cleveland. She was then placed on thioridazine 50 mg hs. On 4 Apr 91 she complained of fatigue on thioridazine 50 mg hs. Speech pause analysis revealed: balance = 52.42%, synchrony = 40.00%, [+] = 14.95%, [-] = 57.04%, [−] = 24.62% (Figure 1). Competence was reduced in both hemispheres, more so on the right. Thioridazine was reduced to 25 mg hs and on 16 May fatigue was less, balance = 50.20%, synchrony = 16.67%, [+] = 11.08%, [-] = 5.16%, [−] = 2.23%; reduced competence limited to the right hemisphere was less marked compared with 4 Apr. She complained of feeling "nervous" and thioridazine was increased to 35 mg hs. On 13 Jun she reported feeling "very calm," balance = 45.18%, synchrony = 80.00%, [+] = 5.54%, [-] = 6.33%, [−] = 1.28%, and no lateralized incompetence could be demonstrated (Figure 2). There were no recurrences of the oculogyric crisis and hallucinations.

These data illustrate application of longitudinal monitoring in the treatment of disruptions of asymmetric brain functions in schizophrenia (Crowe & Kuttner, 1991; Friedman, 1991h). Reduction of thioridazine may have improved her left hemisphere competence and mood measurements by modulating dopamine in the left dorsal

FIGURE 1

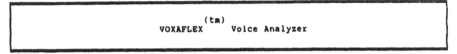

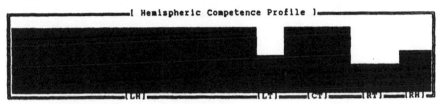

Record: [R] G   B   Ln In dialogue   at 16:52 on 04 Apr 91
    with [L] Ernest Friedman   Elapsed time was: 03:26

Indices: Mood: (+) = 14.95% (-) = 57.04% (--) = 24.62% Comm = NSD
        Balance = 52.42% Synchro = 40.00% Transit = 82.35% Bond = 2.36%

                        Filename is BGFE9140.4X1

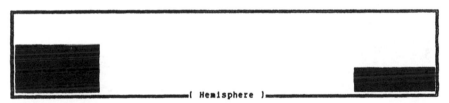

For additional Information contact: VOXAFLEX   Phone: (216) 681-5200
1831 Forest Hills Blvd, East Cleveland, OH 44112-4313 FAX:(216) 368-3186

prefrontal cortex (Friedman, 1990d; Pettegrew et al., 1991). This method may be utilized to detect the neuroleptic threshold (Bitter et al., 1991) to reduce risk of short and long-term adverse effects of psychotropic medication. It also may be utilized to monitor do-paminergic stimulation reducing cognitive processing speed (Poewe et al., 1991) in studies of normal brain function in aging and in other major categories of psychiatric disease, such as anxiety and mood disorders (Guze, 1991).

Speech timing as an objective guide to the prevention of side effects of serotonergic drugs is presented in the following case presentation:

FIGURE 2

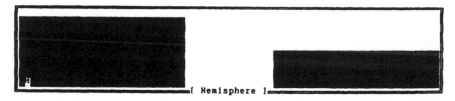

```
                            (tm)
            VOXAFLEX        Voice Analyzer
```

```
Record: [R] G                B       in dialogue           at 16:26 on 13 Jun 91
  with  [L] Ernest Friedman                          Elapsed time was: 05:15

Indices:    Mood:  (+) = 5.54%     (-) = 6.33%     (--) = 1.28%
                   Balance = 45.18%  Synchro = 80.00%  Bond = 31.73%

                   Filename is BGFE9161.3X0
```

```
For additional information contact:     VOXAFLEX      Phone: (216) 681-5200
1831 Forest Hills Blvd, East Cleveland, OH 44112-4313  FAX:(216) 368-3106
```

A 55 year old male (C.H.) developed akathisia in early 1990 when treated with fluoxetine 20 mg qd requiring stopping the drug. On 2 Aug 90 prior to reinstituting fluoxetine, mania [+] = 6.71%, depression [-] = 13.21% and very depressed [−] was 6.67%. The left-hemisphere showed incompetence (upper left bar) and the right-hemisphere was underproductive (lower right bar). In April 91, he was restarted on fluoxetine 5 mg qd and by 23 May showed [+] = 4.30%, [-] = 24.81%, and [−] = NSD. Right-hemisphere competence and productivity were less than ideal although the patient felt he was doing much better. Fluoxetine was increased on 23 May to 7.5 mg qd and by 30 May he said he felt the dose was "just right": [+] = 2.52%, [-] = 5.15%, [−] = 2.56%; the 7.5 mg qd fluoxetine dose was continued.

The detection of switches into mania at night and longitudinal monitoring of treatment response are demonstrated in the following case illustration:

A 62 year old male professional (A.G.) was treated elsewhere for two years with molindone for paranoid delusions with marginal benefit. His guarded manner made interviewing difficult. Evaluation on 30 Jun 90 revealed paranoid delusions without mania; [+] = 30.07%, [-] = 32.53%, [−] = 9.16%. In contrast, monitoring by telephone during accentuation of paranoid delusions after 9 PM on 2 Jul 90, demonstrated [+] = 13.98%, [-] = 5.58%, [−] = NSD (not sufficient data), and reduced right-hemisphere competence and productivity, represented in the right upper and lower bars, respectively. These subtle changes were difficult to detect clinically because of his hypervigilance. Standard psychological testing administered in the afternoon diagnosed Paranoid Delusional Disorder but not Bipolar Mood Disorder. He was stabilized on thiothixene 2 mg hs and lithium carbonate 450 mg bid, attaining a serum lithium level of 0.9 meq/l; by 18 May 91, competence and productivity of brain functions were optimal; [+] = 15.22%, [-] = 6.48%, and [−] = NSD. Because of hand tremor, a thiothixene holiday was attempted while maintaining the lithium which resulted in the recurrence on 26 May 91 of paranoid and somatic delusions, accelerated speech rate and a moderate reduction compared with July 2, 1990, of interhemispheric synchrony, right-hemisphere competence and productivity; [+] = 20.59%, [-] = NSD, [−] = NSD. Thiothixene was restarted and by 28 May 91, paranoid delusions were in partial remission and competence quickly returned. Balance improved but synchrony decreased, and the manic scale was elevated: [+] = 31.22%. Residual somatic preoccupation was present on 10 Jun; early and late afternoon comparison on 10 Jun 91 demonstrated decreased synchrony but increased balance; diurnal mood variation was similar to 30 Jun/2 Jul 90: 10 Jun 91 2:00 pm [+] = 21.69%, [-] = 32.06%, [−] = 8.96%; 5:47 pm [+] = 16.87%, [-] = 4.85%, [−] = NSD suggesting evaluation of mood variation monitored by LP and right hemisphere competence monitored by SP.

Treatment of depression in a person with dyslexia is demonstrated by the following example:

A 20 year old dyslexic male college student (E.L.) who had been treated with methylphenidate as a child for hyperactivity, was evaluated on 24 May 1990 for depression with suicidal ideation. There was a history of autism in a paternal uncle. Marked decrease in left-hemisphere competence was accompanied by balance = 6.66%, synchrony = 56.67%, [+] = 3.36%, [-] = 75.49%, [−] = 9.21%. Fluoxetine was increased gradually to 100 mg qd and by 13 Oct 1990 left-hemisphere competence had improved somewhat, balance = 74.47%, synchrony = 50.00%, [+] = 7.26%, [-] = 2.89%, [−] = NSD. An attempt was made to taper the dose and by 21 Feb 1991 on 40 mg qd of fluoxetine left-hemisphere incompetence was again evident, balance = 6.90%, synchrony = 66.67%, [+] = 8.35%, [-] = 55.87%, [−] 4.29. The 100 mg qd dosage regimen was gradually reinstituted and by 9 Apr 1991 left-hemisphere competence had returned to its previous modest level, balance = 77.48%, synchrony = 83.34%, [+] = 11.26%, [-] = NSD, [−] = NSD. He attended special classes for his dyslexia which was not significantly benefitted by fluoxetine. However, he reported that his concentration in general in addition to his mood had improved since he had begun the fluoxetine regimen.

These findings support the role of the left dorsal anterolateral prefrontal cortex in depression (Friedman, 1990d), and of inefficient allocation of a circumscribed left hemisphere region to verbal processing in poor readers (Flowers et al., 1991).

FUTURE RESEARCH DIRECTIONS

The role of speech pause monitoring in the diagnosis and treatment of mood disorders can be tested in psychiatric practice by using remote data collection to detect previously undiagnosed switches into mania at night. It can be utilized to determine the frequency of mood cycling and amplitude of diurnal and reverse diurnal mood rhythms. Lateralized brain functions in panic disorder associated with coronary risk and mood disorder, and biofeedback of coronary prone behavior all need additional research studies. Reduced competence, efficiency and speed of brain functions may be examined in attention deficit disorder associated with mood disorder in school populations. Participatory matching can be examined in family therapy, organizational development, and in teacher-student interactions. The evaluation of prefrontal brain competence in schizophrenics as a way to predict medication response (Friedman, 1991) can be examined further. These methods have also been used to detect neuroleptic thresholds (Bitter, 1991) for schizophrenics and this needs further investigation to predict best possible medication doses and thus minimize side-effects.

SOFTWARE AVAILABILITY

The VOXAFLEX voice monitor, software, and instructions are available for $18,500 through: VOXAFLEX, 1821 Forest Hills Blvd., East Cleveland, OH 44112-4313, (216) 681-5200 or Fax (216) 368-3106.

REFERENCES

Altshuler, L.L., Conrad, A., Hauser, P, Ximing, L., Guze, B. H., Denikoff, K., Tourtellotte, W. & Post, R. (1991). Reduction of temporal lobe volume in bipolar disorder: a preliminary report of magnetic resonance imaging (letter). Archives of General Psychiatry, 48, 482-483.

Bakhtin, M.M. (1986). Speech Genres and Other Late Essays. Austin: University of Texas Press.

Barton, A., Bowie, J. & Ebmeier, K. (1990). Low plasma iron status and akathisia. Journal of Neurology, Neurosurgery, and Psychiatry, 53, 671-674.

Bernstein, B. (1962). Linguistic codes, hesitation phenomena and intelligence. Language and Speech, 5, 31-48.

Bitter, I., Volavka, J. & Scheurer, J. (1991). The concept of the neuroleptic threshold: an update. Journal of Clinical Psychopharmacology, 11, 28-33.

Blondin, J.P. and Waked, E.G., (1991). Cardiovascular responses, performance, and mood in heart rate reactive individuals during a challenging cognitive task. Personality and Individual Differences, 12:825-834.

Boone, K.B., Ananth, J., Philpott, L., Kaur, A. & Djenderedjian, A. (1991). Neuropsychological characteristics of nondepressed adults with obsessive-compulsive disorder. Neuropsychiatry, Neuropsychology & Behavioral Neurology, 4, 96-109.

Braunig, P. (1990). Switch processes and rapid cycling in bipolar affective disorders, cycloid psychoses and nonsystematic schizophrenia. Psychopathology, 23, 291-302.

Brenowitz, E.A. (1991). Altered perception of species-specific song by female birds after lesions of a forebrain nucleus. Science, 251, 303-305.

Brown, T.R.E., Glen, S.E. & White, T. (1987). Low serum iron status and akathisia. Lancet i:1234-1236.

Brown, V.J. & Robbins, T.W. (1991). Simple and choice reaction time performance following unilateral striatal dopamine depletion in the rat: impaired motor readiness but preserved response preparation. Brain, 114, 513-525.

Bunney, W.E. Jr. & Hartmann, E.L. (1965). Study of a patient with 48 hour manic-depressive cycles. Archives of General Psychiatry, 12, 611-618.

Bunney, W.E. Jr., Murphy, D.L., Goodwin, F.K. & Borge, G.F. (1972a). The "switch process" in manic-depressive illness: I. A systematic study of sequential behavioral changes. Archives of General Psychiatry, 27, 295-302.

Bunney, W.E. Jr., Murphy, D.L., Goodwin, F.K., House, K.M. & Gordon, E.K. (1972b). The "switch process" in manic-depressive illness: II. Relationship to catecholamines, REM sleep, and drugs. Archives of General Psychiatry, 27, 304-309.

Bunney, W.E. Jr., Murphy, D.L. & Goodwin, F.K. (1972c). The "switch process" in manic-depressive illness: III. Theoretical implications. Archives of General Psychiatry, 27, 312-317.

Christenson, G.A., Popkin, M.K., Mackenzie, T.B. & Realmuto, G.M. (1991). Lithium treatment of chronic hair pulling. Journal of Clinical Psychiatry, 52, 116-120.

Cooke, P. (1991). The cried until they could not see. New York Times Magazine, June 23.

Crowe, C.F. & Kuttner, M. (1991). Differences between schizophrenia and the schizophrenia-like, psychosis of temporal lobe epilepsy: support for the two-process view of schizophrenia. Neuropsychiatry, Neuropsychology & Behavioral Neurology, 4, 127-135.

Crown, C.L. & Feldstein, S. (1991). The perception of speech rate from the sound-silence patterns of monologues. Journal of Psycholinguistic Research, 20, 47-63.

Crystal, T.H. & House, A.H. (1982). Segmental durations in connected speech signals: preliminary results. Journal of the Acoustical Society of America. 72, 705-716.

Csernansky, J.G., Murphy, G.M. and Faustman, W.O. (1991). Limbic/mesolimbic connections and the pathogenesis of schizophrenia. Biological Psychiatry 30:383-400.

Flowers, D.L., Wood, F.B. & Naylor, C.E. (1991). Regional cerebral blood flow correlates of language processes in reading disability. Archives of Neurology, 48, 637-643.

Fontana, A.F., Rosenberg, R.L., Burg, M.M., Kerns, R.D. & Colonese, K.L. (1990). Type A Behavior and self-referencing: interactive risk factors? Journal of Social Behavior and Personality, 5, 215-232.

Friedman, E.H. & Sanders, G.G. (1988). Speech pattern analysis. In J. G. Webster (Ed.), Encyclopedia of Medical Devices and Instrumentation. New York: Wiley, pp. 2642-2652.

Friedman, E.H. (1989a). Speech timing of integrative brain functions (Abstract #8). Neuroscience: Integrative Functions; The First Annual Bristol-Myers Symposium on Neuroscience Research. The Johns Hopkins Medical Institutions, Baltimore, October 11-12.

Friedman, E.H. (1989b). Participatory matching (letter). American Journal of Psychiatry, 146, 1650.

Friedman, E.H. (1990a). VOXAFLEX speech pause time monitor (software survey section). Journal of Child Psychology and Psychiatry, 31, I.Friedman, E.H. (1990b). Letter to the editor. Journal of Psychosomatic Research, 34, 591.

Friedman, E.H. (1990c). Temporal lobe in schizophrenia (letter). British Journal of Psychiatry, 157, 784-785.

Friedman, E.H. (1990d). Akathisia (letter). British Journal of Psychiatry, 156, 285.

Friedman, E.H. & Benson, D.F. (1990e). Hesitation (letter & reply). Neuropsychiatry, Neuropsychology & Behavioral Neurology, 3, 236-237.

Friedman, E.H., Guthrie, S. & Grunhaus, L. (1990f). Fluoxetine and stuttering (letter and reply). Journal of Clinical Psychiatry, 51, 310-311.

Friedman, E.H. (1991a). Temporal processing (letter). Journal of Learning Disabilities, 24, 260.

Friedman, E.H. (1991b). On "Consultation-liaison in child psychiatry and the evolution of pediatric psychiatry" (letter). Psychosomatics, 32, 116.

Friedman, E.H. (1991c). The role of the right hemisphere in fluoxetine-induced bradycardia and syncope (letter). Journal of Clinical Psychiatry, 52, 138-139.

Friedman, E.H. (1991d). Electroconvulsive therapy for a depressed patient with global aphasia (letter). Psychosomatics, 32, 237.

Friedman, E.H. (1991e). Speech pauses and diagnosis (letter). Journal of Clinical Psychiatry, 52, 181-182.

Friedman, E.H. (1991f). Letter to the editor. Social Science & Medicine, 32, 1317-1318.

Friedman, E.H. (1991g). Biogenic amines in tardive dyskinesia (letter). Journal of Nervous and Mental Diseases, 179, 304-305.

Friedman, E.H. (1991h). Cerebral atrophy in schizophrenia (letter to the editor). Neuropsychiatry, Neuropsychology & Behavioral Neurology, 4, 169-170.

Friedman, E.H. & Jacobs, S. (1991i). Anxiety disorders during acute bereavement (letter and reply). Journal of Clinical Psychiatry, 52, 241.

Friedman, E.H. & Robinson, R.G. (1991j). Speech hesitation pauses as markers for mood disorder in stroke patients? (letter and reply). Journal of Clinical Psychiatry, 52, 140.

Fries, W. & Swihart, A.A. (1990). Disturbance of rhythm sense following right hemisphere damage. Neuropsychologia, 28, 1317-1323.

Gambert, S.R., Gupta, K.L., Friedman, E.H., Aronson, M.K., Ooi, W.L. Frishman, W. & Masur, D.M. (1991). Women and dementia (letters and reply). Neurology, 41, 461-462.

Gilley, D.W., Wilson, R.S., Bennett, D.A., Stebbins, G.T., Bernard, B.A., Whalen, M.E. & Fox, J.H. (1991). Cessation of driving and unsafe motor vehicle operation by dementia patients. Archives of Internal Medicine, 151, 941-946.

Goldman-Eisler, F. (1968). Psycholinguistics: experiments in spontaneous speech. London & New York: Academic Press.

Goodwin, F.K. & Jamison K.R. (1990). Manic-depressive illness. New York: Oxford University Press.

Guscott, R. & Grof, P. (1991). The clinical meaning of refractory depression: a review for the clinician. American Journal of Psychiatry, 148, 695-704.

Guze, B.H. (1991). Magnetic resonance spectroscopy: a technique for functional brain imaging. Archives of General Psychiatry, 48, 572-574.

Halliday, T.R. & Houston, A.I. (1991). How long will newts wait? An experiment to test an assumption of a causal model of the courtship of the male smooth newt, Triturus V. Vulgaris. Behaviour, 116, 278-291.

Heyman, A., Fillenbaum, G., Prosnitz, B., Raiford, K., Burchett, B. & Clark, C. (1991). Estimated prevalence of dementia among elderly black and white community residents. Archives of Neurology, 48, 594-598.

Hyde, A.P. (1990). Varying presentations of bipolar II disorder make diagnosis difficult. The Psychiatric Times, October, pp. 56-58.

Isabella, R.A. & Belsky, J. (1991). Interactional synchrony and the origins of infant-mother attachment: a replication study. Child Development, 62, 373-384.

Jaffe. J. and Feldstein, S., (1970). Rhythms of Dialogue. New York and London: Academic Press.

Kruger, H.-P. (1989). Speech chronemics — a hidden dimension of speech. Theoretical background, measurement and clinical validity. Pharmacopsychiatry, 22, 5-12.

Liotti, M., Sava, D., Rizzolati, G. & Caffarra, P. (1991). Differential hemispheric asymmetries in depression and anxiety: a reaction-time study. Biological Psychiatry, 29, 887-899.

Marler, P. (1991). Song-learning behavior: the interface with neuroethology. Trends in Neuroscience, 14, 199-206.

Mizukawa, R., Ishiguro, S., Takada, H., Kishimoto, A., Ogura, C. & Hazama, H. (1991). Long-term observation of a manic-depressive patient with rapid cycles. Biological Psychiatry, 29, 671-678.

Modell, J.G, Mountz, J.M., Curtis, G.C. & Greden, J.F. (1989). Neurophysiologic dysfunction in basal ganglia/limbic striatal and thalamocortical circuits as a pathogenetic mechanism of obsessive compulsive disorder. Journal of Neuropsychiatry, 1, 27-36.

Mulcahy, D., Purcell, H. & Fox, K. (1991). Should we get up in the morning? Observations on circadian variation in cardiac events. British Heart Journal, 65, 299-301.

Natelson, B.H., Tapp, W.N., Drastal, S., Scares, R. & Ottenweller, JG. (1991). Hamsters with coronary vasospasm are at increased risk from stress. Psychosomatic Medicine, 53, 322-331.

Nemes, Z.C., Rotrosen, J., Angrist, B., Peselow, E. & Schoentag, R. (1991). Serum iron levels and akathisia. Biological Psychiatry, 29, 411-413.

Nottebohm, F. (1991). Reassessing the mechanisms and origins of vocal learning in birds. Trends in Neuroscience, 14, 206-211.

O'Boyle, M. W., Bormann, L. & Harts, K. (1990). How knowledge of the song influences the matching of "melodies" to rhythm sequences tapped in the left and right palms. Cortex, 26, 639-642.

Pascual-Leone, A., Gates, J.R. & Dhuna, A. (1991). Induction of speech arrest and counting errors with rapid-rate transcranial magnetic stimulation. Neurology, 41, 697-702.

Petitto, L.A. & Marentette, P.J. (1991). Babbling in the manual mode: evidence for the ontogeny of language. Science, 251, 1493-1496.

Pettegrew, J.W., Keshavan, M.S., Panchalingam, K., Strychor, S., Kaplan, D.B., Tretta, M.G. & Allen, M. (1991). Alterations in brain high-energy phosphate and membrane phospholipid metabolism in first-episode, drug-naive schizophrenics: a pilot study of the dorsal prefrontal cortex by in vivo phosphorus 31 nuclear magnetic resonance spectroscopy. Archives of General Psychiatry, 48, 563-568.

Pindzola, R.H. (1990). Dysfluency characteristics of aged, normal-speaking black and white males. Journal of Fluency Disorders, 15, 235-243.

Poewe, W., Berger, W., Benke, Th. & Schelosky, L. (1991). High-speed memory scanning in Parkinson's disease: adverse effects of levodopa. Annals of Neurology, 29, 670-673.

Pollard, C.A., Ibe, I.O., Krojanker, D.N., Kitchen, A.D., Bronson, S.S. & Flynn, T. (1991). Clomipramine treatment of trichotillomania: a follow-up report on four cases. Journal of Clinical Psychiatry, 52, 128-130.

Rammsayer, T. (1990). Temporal discrimination in schizophrenic and affective disorders: evidence for a dopamine-dependent internal clock. International Journal of Neuroscience, 53, 111-120.

Robin, D.A., Tranel, D. & Damasio, H. (1990). Auditory perception of temporal and spectral events in patients with focal left and right cerebral lesions. Brain and Language, 39, 539-555.

Safire, W. (1991). Impregnating the pause. The New York Times Magazine, June 16.

Savithri, S.R. (1988). Speech and hearing science in ancient India: a review of Sanskrit literature. Journal of Communication Disorders, 21, 271-317.

Schou, M. & Weeke, A. (1988). Did manic-depressive patients who committed suicide receive prophylactic or continuation treatment at the time? British Journal of Psychiatry, 153, 324-327.

Silva, L.R., Amital, Y. & Connors, B.W. (1991). Intrinsic oscillations of neocortex generated by layer 5 pyramidal neurons. Science, 251, 432-435.

Stagno, S.J., Naugle, R.I., Roca, C. & Estes, M. (1990). Language disturbance and progressive multifocal leukoencephalopathy. Neuropsychiatry, Neuropsychology and Behavioral Neurology, 3, 283-290).

Steele, J. (1779). Prosodia Rationalis. Reprinted by Hildesheim & New York 1971: Georg Olms Verlag.

Szamosi, G. (1986). The Twin Dimensions: Inventing Time and Space. New York: Wiley.

Tallmer, J., Scherwitz, L., Chesney, M., Hecker, M., Hunkeler, E., Serwitz, J. & Hughes, G. (1990). Selection, training, and quality control of Type A interviewers in a prospective study of young adults. Journal of Behavioral Medicine. 13, 449-466.

Taylor, R. (1991). A lot of "excitement" about neurodegeneration: suggestive data indicate that "excitotoxicity" could play a role in Alzheimer's and in Parkinson's. Science, 252, 1380-1381.

Welford, A.T. (1988). Reaction time, speed of performance and age. Annals of the New York Academy of Sciences, 515, 1-17.

Welkowitz, J., Bond, R.N. & Zelano, J. (1990). An automated system for the analyses of temporal speech patterns: description of the hardware and software. Journal of Communication Disorders, 23, 347-364.

Zielinski, C.M., Taylor, M.A. & Juzwin, K.R. (1991). Neuropsychological deficits in obsessive-compulsive disorder. Neuropsychiatry, Neuropsychology & Behavioral Neurology, 4, 110-126.

A Knowledge Based System
for Assisting in Differential Diagnosis
of Chemically Dependent/
Mentally Ill Patients

Robert John Bischoff

KEYWORDS. Computer assisted diagnosis, mental health software, substance abuse, computerized patient testing

SUMMARY. This paper discusses the use of Knowledge Base 2.1, a computer program that administers a response dependent, structured interview to evaluate the presence of psychiatric disorders within the chemical dependency treatment setting. The writer reviews the problems commonly encountered when conducting clinical interviews, psychometric examinations and differentially diagnosing psychiatric disorders within this special population. Knowledge Base 2.1 utilizes combined computer techniques of rule driven logic, pattern matching, and an original algorithm that accomplishes a "real time restandardization" of the complete database. With each administration, restandardization is implemented in an effort to adequately consider the effects of chemical dependency on psychological test performance and normative information regarding symptoms. Knowledge Base 2.1 also functions as a research tool inasmuch as all patient responses to this structured interview are permanently stored in computer files for ongoing analysis.

INTRODUCTION

We review the conception, development and implementation of a knowledge based system for assisting in differential diagnosis of chemically dependent/ mentally ill patients, herein to be referred to

Robert John Bischoff, PhD, 10601 South De Anza Boulevard, Cupertino, CA 95014.

as the Dual Diagnosis Knowledge Base or KB 2.1 program, an original, computerized, screening tool for use in the assessment of psychiatric disorders within the chemical dependency population. The program utilizes innovative programming techniques to investigate organic brain dysfunction, level of withdrawal symptoms, anxiety, mood disorders, eating disorders, gambling, sexual trauma and deviations, suicide indicators, denial of disease, and personality disorders.

TRADITIONAL EVALUATION

The normal thorough assessment process including documentation of the completed interview and test batteries for both neuropsychological difficulties and "dual diagnosis" (psychiatrically disordered patients within the chemically dependent patient population) may involve as much as half of the available clinical time. Additionally, in the past decade of test administration, at O'Connor Hospital Inpatient Chemical Dependency treatment unit, (O'Connor Hospital 1990) certain characteristic scores have emerged from the instruments used. For example, standardized depression measures have yielded a consistent mild to moderate level of depression for patients who were beyond the detoxification stage of their inpatient treatment. While depression inventories were helpful in identifying significantly depressed patients, it addressed only one clinical feature. It was still necessary to administer, hand score, and record the results for each patient who required screening. There were also some unique issues that consistently emerged for persons who had abused alcohol or other chemicals including a variety of compulsive behaviors, anxiety, mood disturbances, sexual traumas and abuses, eating disorders, a host of personality disorders and multiple neurological deficits.

RATIONALE FOR COMPUTER APPROACHES

Because of differences in levels of pathology or acuity across settings or populations, a need for norms for these similar but different populations is indicated.

Prior structured clinical interviews conducted by this author and selected psychometrics, including the Minnesota Multiphasic Personality Inventory, for use with this population had addressed these areas quite thoroughly as long as issues of set and setting were factored into the interpretation; however, time constraints given the increasing flow of patients requiring assessment called for a more efficient approach to serve patients and staff needs.

Computers are adeptly designed for well structured and repetitive tasks with a certain constancy of features such as the present problem. However, despite the personal computer explosion of the early 1980's, proliferation of a wide variety of applications software for the general public and appearance of computerized software in psychological publishing house catalogues for specific testing and analysis of test results, there is no evidence of any software available for assessment of psychiatric illness in the chemically dependent with the exception of neuropsychiatric assessment by computer. To date, the use of computers relative to the chemical dependency field of study has been focused mainly in the areas of education (Brown, Carlson 1990; Brown, Byrne 1990; Brown, Carter, Gordon 1987), evaluation of physiological processes (Beresford, Low, Hall, Adduci, Goggang 1982; Johnson, Adinoff, Bisserbe, Martin 1986; Carlen, Penn, Fornazzoni, Bennett 1986), chemical dependency detection through a variety of methods (Beresford, Blow, Hill, Singer, Lucey 1990; Barry, Fleming 1990; Paperny, Aono, Lehman, Hammar, Risser 1990; Anderson 1987; Bernhardt, Ferraio 1988) and as previously noted, neuropsychological evaluation (Acker 1980; John, Prichep, Fridman, Easton 1988; MacDonell, Skinner, Glen 1987). And while there have been considerable advances in computer use in the area of psychiatric diagnosis (Greist, Klein, Erdman, Jefferson 1983), there is a lack of software that might be useful to cover the myriad comorbid diagnoses that are normally present for the chemically dependent.

Furthermore, because of clinical features which are typical within the chemically dependent population that would be considered statistically significant or abnormal for even a psychiatric patient based standardization population, symptom specific tests such as those tests which evaluate for depression, provide initially misleading results. This could render 'canned' report generators completely useless for this special population.

Through 1989, there were no computerized instruments in general use which would address clinicians needs for evaluating psychiatric problems in the chemically dependent.

COMPUTER PROGRAM DEVELOPMENT

The current program which is written in Turbo Pascal 6.0 (TM), and provides not only a structured interview similar to the one that I was performing almost daily in my clinical practice, but also produces local normative information for use within the structured interview logic as well as in calculating the diagnostic outcome.

This program is unique in its ability to simultaneously evaluate for a wide variety of psychiatric problems which are often found within the chemically dependent population, perform a real time "restandardization-on-the-fly" of the patient population database and compare the currently tested patient to these findings.

This "restandardization-on-the-fly" not only solves the problem encountered by using instruments which are permanently bound to their original standardization populations, but allows for a much more dynamic and discreet evaluation within the specific population. For example, upon examination of the clinical records maintained by this author, it is noteworthy that the mean score for reported symptoms of organic dysfunction is higher for the O'Connor Hospital inpatient chemical dependency population than its outpatient program counterpart in San Jose, California. While this may seem to follow common sense as well as partly validate the need for inpatient treatment for some patients, it also underscores the need for local norms of testing information. Further, the tedious task of tracking this test score information and doing the recalculation needed for T score comparisons is done completely and automatically by the KB 2.1 program.

One of the major problems with conducting research using clinical interviews and test instruments is not only the collection of demographic information, but the need for someone to enter this information into a computer program which ultimately performs the analysis. A major feature of KB 2.1 is the presentation of a data collection screen as an initial portion of the screening process which is then written to a disk file for later analysis as well as in the high suicide risk profile. In fact, all information entered by the patient is written to disk files, including every individual keystroke. This permanent record of responses allows for tremendous flexibility in terms of future research that one might wish to conduct. Future versions of KB 2.1 will exploit this feature.

STATISTICAL BASIS FOR BRANCHING LOGIC

When KB 2.1 was first being developed, cutting scores were based solely upon clinical hunches and experience, since the database was very small ($N < 50$). The structured interview was designed to cover all areas, which in this author's experience were problematic to the individual in early recovery from chemical dependency. The interview questions were weighted and these weights were used to determine whether more questions were to be asked or if a particular diagnosis might be applicable. Further, if some of the questions were answered in a particular direction, that event would trigger other questions to deepen the inquiry. An example of cumulative weights deepening the inquiry is evidenced in the initial inquiry regarding symptoms of anxiety. Should the patient answer any of three of an initial six questions regarding anxiety indicating pathology, then the additional twelve questions are presented. An example of one question triggering a deepened inquiry is typified by the patient answering yes to the question, "Have you been feeling like or thinking about killing yourself recently?" An affirmative answer launches a very structured set of questions which attempt to define the patients's level of risk. This process yields useful clinical information for each patient, which has been continually evaluated and assessed for efficacy and accuracy. With the steady increase of patients within the database ($N > 100$), the "restandardization-on-the-fly" feature took precedence over the original cutting scores and significantly increased the power of the instrument. Questions about what might be normal for a patient within this specific population for a particular psychiatric feature would be evident, such as the problem of clinical features of depression previously mentioned.

When the patient has completed approximately two thirds of the structured interview, the instrument activates the statistical section which then sums the patient's scores, calculates means, standard deviations and computes the patients' T scores using the disk based database. After deriving this information, T score driven logic is implemented to determine if further questioning is indicated and if so, in what specific areas. For example, if a patient's T scores are abnormally low or high (T score cutoffs of 40 and 60 respectively) in a specific area, KB 2.1 goes about asking more questions in an effort to 'understand' why this has occurred. Issues of impaired reading ability, misunderstanding of question content and intent, gross organic difficulties and severely oppositional attitudes are considered in attempting to evaluate the patient's performance. The use of absurd questions tests for possible impaired reading skills, poor reality testing, or attitudinal problems. Further, the patient answering in the affirmative to the items portraying confusion, lack of understanding, inadequate functioning or a clearly hostile or negative attitude towards the interview process helps to qualify the patient's KB 2.1 results and diagnostic statements. The program then moves to a section which evaluates the likelihood of psychiatric problems being present for this patient based upon total outcome.

DIAGNOSIS GENERATION

A combination of DSM-III(R) (APA 1987) criteria and the patient's T scores is used as a basis for identifying possible secondary psychiatric diagnosis. In the differential diagnosis section of KB 2.1, not only does the DSM-III(R) criteria need to be met for a particular diagnosis, but the Tscore for that diagnosis variable needs to be significant for the test population ($T > 60$) as well.

The KB 2.1 software also can be configured to launch or administer other applications from within itself. That is, if the clinician has an application software package which they had been using to test for depression, eating disorders, or other clinical features, KB 2.1 can be configured to run this software as a routine matter only if certain rules are satisfied. This allows the clinician to continue to use other existing software with which they are already familiar and comfortable.

Of the numerous possible findings generated by KB 2.1, suicide potential is noteworthy. In an effort to alert the clinician to the possibility of suicide for a particular patient, there is a high suicide profile embedded within the instrument which is designed to detect the high risk patient. This high risk profile is based upon age, employment status, availability of emotional supports, and other cogent factors. The more extensive inquiry into suicide potential is triggered automatically if the patient openly acknowledges suicidal intent or history and is triggered indirectly by the patient's demographic and other pertinent information noted above. If a patient's scoring is significant, a no harm contract is automatically generated along with the two disk files which contain the findings and diagnostic information and is printed when the ancillary printing program is activated.

PROGRAM INFORMATION

In addition to the disk files noted earlier with regard to future research efforts there are two disk files containing the findings, PATIENT.FIL and WORK.FIL. Both files are printed by an ancillary program called HARDCOPY.EXE. The PATIENT.FIL contains the specific findings in each of the interview areas, a summary of the local normative data, diagnostic findings for Axis I and II of DSM-III(R), a critical items listing and finally additional clinical findings that are generated only if certain criteria are met during the interview process. The PATIENT.FIL output is in a format that makes it highly suitable for inclusion within the patient's chart; a feature that alone is of great value given the need for thorough documentation of patient treatment by managed health care and other reviewers. The second file, WORK.FIL, is a work sheet for the clinician. In addition to most of the information contained in the PATIENT.FIL, this file contains information which is highly speculative and may warrant further investigation by the clinician. This file may be particularly useful for record keeping and consultation by the clinician long after the medical chart has been forwarded to medical records.

All questions contained within KB 2.1 were designed by this author based upon a decade of clinical experience in the assessment of the chemically dependent patient with the exception of the question series evaluating for the possible presence of personality disorders. The whole of these questions where developed by Goldberg, (1989) and are contained herein with his express permission.

KB 2.1 was designed to facilitate a thorough screening of the chemically dependent patient in both inpatient and outpatient settings and to promote painless research. It is designed for use by a clinician who is interested in the development of local normative information on their specific populations. It is currently appropriate for use in either an inpatient or outpatient setting for patients over the age of eighteen and can be easily administered by nursing or clerical staff.

SOFTWARE AVAILABILITY

KB 2.1 is approximately 370K bytes in size and requires an IBM PC/XT/AT (TM) or compatible computer with 640K of memory. KB 2.1 is still under development with additional innovative features which will be addressed in a later paper. The program will be available commercially at a later time.

REFERENCES

Acker, W. (1980). A microcomputer administered neuropsychological assessment system for use with chronic alcoholics. Substance Alcohol Actions Misuse, 1(5-6), 545-50.

Anderson R.V. (1987). Computerization of a chemical dependency assessment. Minnesota Medical, Dec, 70(12), 697-9.

American Psychiatric Association. Diagnostic and Statistical Manual of Mental Disorders (3rd ed.). Washington D.C.: American Psychiatric Association, 1987.

Barry K.L., Fleming M.F. (1990). Computerized administration of alcoholism screening tests in a primary care setting. Journal of American Board of Family Practice, Apr-Jun, 3(2), 93-8.

Beresford T.P., Blow F.C., Hill E., Singer K., Lucey M.R. (1990). Comparison of CAGE questionnaire and computer-assisted laboratory profiles in screening for covert alcoholism. Lancet Aug 25, 336(8713), 482-5.

Beresford T., Low D., Hall R.C., Adduci R., Goggans F. (1982). A computerized biochemical profile for the detection of alcoholism. Psychosomatics, Jul, 23(7), 713-4, 719-20.

Bernhardt A.J., Ferraio N.L., (1988). Description and evaluation of the Minnesota Assessment of Chemical Health software package. Employee Assistance Quarterly, Vol 4(1), 1-18.

Brown R.L., Byrne K. (1990). Computer-assisted curriculum for medical students on early diagnosis of substance abuse. Family Medicine, Jul-Aug, 22(4), 288-92.

Brown R.L., Carlson B.L. (1990). Early diagnosis of substance abuse: evaluation of a course of computer-assisted instruction. Medical Education, Sep, 24(5), 438-46.

Brown R.L., Carter W.B., Gordon M.J. (1987). Diagnosis of alcoholism in a simulated patient encounter by primary care physicians. Journal of Family Practice, 25(3), 259-64.

Carlen P.L., Penn R.D., Fornazzari L., Bennett J. et al. (1986). Computerized tomographic scan assessment of alcoholic brain damage and its potential reversibility. Annual Meeting of the Research Society on Alcoholism: Imaging research in alcoholism. Alcoholism: Clinical & Experimental Research, Jun, 10(3), 226-32.

Greist, J. H., Klein, M.H., Erdman, H.P., & Jefferson, J.W. (1983). Computers and Psychiatric Diagnosis. Psychiatric Annals, 13(10), 785, 789-92.

John E.R., Prichep L.S., Fridman J., Easton P., (1988). Neurometrics: computer-assisted differential diagnosis of brain dysfunctions. Science, Jan 8, 239(4836), 162-9.

Johnson J.L., Adinoff B., Bisserbe J, Martin P.R. et al. (1986). Assessment of alcoholism-related organic brain syndromes with positron emission tomography. Annual Meeting of the Research Society on Alcoholism: Imaging research in alcoholism. Alcoholism: Clinical & Experimental Research, Jun, 10(3), 237-40.

MacDonell L.E., Skinner F.K., Glen E.M. (1987). The use of two automated neuropsychological tests, Cogfun and the Perceptual Maze Test, with alcoholics. Alcohol, 22(3), 285-95.

Paperney D.M., Aono J.Y., Lehman R.M., Hammar S.L., Risser J., (1990). Computer-assisted detection and intervention in adolescent high-risk behaviors. Journal of Pediatrics, Mar, 116(3), 456-62.

TRANS:
A PC-Pilot Preprocessor
for Behavioral Health Education

Lynda B. M. Ellis
Paul Welle
Sue V. Petzel

KEYWORDS. Computer assisted instruction, cystic fibrosis, chronic illness, health education

INTRODUCTION

Computer-assisted instruction (CAI) has been used for a number of years to teach concepts used in areas as diverse as elementary arithmetic and care of critically ill patients. Teaching concepts, facts or information are by their very nature relatively straightforward: the fact is given, a situation requiring knowledge of the fact is presented, and a question is asked to determine if the fact is recalled. Answers can be scored and remediation given based on score, facts, or concepts not yet mastered.

Lynda B. M. Ellis, PhD, is Associate Professor in the Division of Health Computer Sciences, Department of Laboratory Medicine and Pathology at the University of Minnesota. Sue V. Petzel, PhD, is a staff psychologist at the Health Psychology Clinic, University of Minnesota, Box 731 UMHC, Minneapolis, MN 55455. The work was supported in part by NIH DER HL37504-02. The address of Lynda B. M. Ellis is Box 511 UMHC, 420 SE Delaware St. Minneapolis, MN 55455.

The authors thank Lily Chen for assistance in lesson development. They also thank Dr. Warren Warwick and the staff of the University of Minnesota Regional Cystic Fibrosis Center for their help with lesson design and evaluation. Write to the author for information regarding software availability.

However, behavioral education attempts to change behavior as well as impart information. Teaching facts or concepts is necessary but not sufficient. Lessons must also motivate behavioral change.

In the early 1980s a research question asked by one author (SP) was "Can computer-assisted instruction be used to teach topics in behavioral health education?" Others have asked similar questions (for a review, see Lambert and Billings, 1991). For example, workers have studied microcomputer use in smoking cessation programs (Burling et al., 1989; Schneider, 1986) and contingency management (Tombari et al., 1985). Multiple hours of CAI lessons on a behavioral topic are required to attempt to compare its use to other methods of behavior modification.

With the support of Dr. Warren Warwick, Director of the University of Minnesota Regional Cystic Fibrosis Center, two of the authors (SP and LE) developed a lesson series to teach coping skills to parents of children with cystic fibrosis. Work began in 1983. The first lesson, an introduction and overview of the expected series, was written in Applesoft Basic(TM) for use on an Apple II microcomputer. The next lesson, written in Apple SuperPILOT(TM), was written in 1985, and subsequently moved to PC Pilot(TM) for use on an IBM PC(TM). Completion of the 11-lesson series required both research funding and development of authoring tools specific to behavioral education.

Behavioral health education, by its very nature, requires more sophisticated CAI authoring tools than most lessons designed only to teach facts or concepts. First, the authors (content experts) are busy health professionals with multiple responsibilities which limit or eliminate time available to master complex lesson authoring systems.

Second, the lessons require individualization. Behavioral therapists do not offer general advice in one-on-one counseling. Rather, for example, they ask clients for their likes and dislikes, details about their family life and support systems or to identify goals they intend to pursue. The therapists then incorporate these into specific suggestions or recommendations for behavioral change. Such personalization requires more complex response processing than typically is used for other types of CAI.

Third, the lessons were to be used by members of the general public, rather than traditional students. Therefore, functions such as sound, graphics and animation are useful to increase the users' interest in lesson content and to focus their attention on learning rather than competing situational/environmental demands. Though not a restriction on the authoring system, the lessons must also be written at a low reading level since the target population has minimal prerequisite level of literacy.

No CAI authoring system now or then could meet all requirements: easy to use and easy to learn to use; permits complex response processing; and permits incorporation of special effects such as sound, graphics, and animation. The response processing and special effects functionalities were most important. PC Pilot(TM) offered them as part of a complete programming language.

The research project to develop and evaluate CAI materials was funded in 1987. One initial priority was the development of TRANS, an easy to learn, easy to use PC Pilot(TM) preprocessor especially designed for behavioral health education.

MATERIALS AND METHODS

PC Pilot(TM), version 2.0, was obtained from the University of Washington, Seattle under site licence to the University of Minnesota. TRANS was written in Microsoft BASIC(TM). CAI lessons were developed and used on an IBM-compatible Zenith EZ-PC(TM) with a 20 Mbyte hard disk drive and monochrome, CGA monitor.

TRANS was evaluated in the development of 11 lessons on coping skills for the parents of children with cystic fibrosis. We determined its ability to do the job and to be used directly by busy health professionals.

RESULTS

TRANS

The TRANS program as developed can take text files saved using the ASCII code (ASCII files) containing lesson text and a few simple formatting codes and produce functional PC-Pilot(TM) code. There is easy addition of PC-Pilot(TM) modules, such as those for graphics, sound, and/or animation. Text is automatically vertical and horizontal centered. There is easy authoring and scoring of multiple choice and true/false questions.

In addition, TRANS automatically allows a user to repeat (backup to) previous screens, stores answers to all questions, permits linking of lesson subsections, assists in lesson standardization, and allows the complex response processing needed to personalize each lesson.

Examples of this response processing are shown in Appendices 1 and 2. Appendix 1 starts with a simple gender query (Is your child a girl or a boy?). This permits the subsequent name question to be personalized (if the child is a girl, the question is "What is her name?"). The questions are asked in this order, not only to permit personalization, but also because some parents think poorly of a computer which needs to ask the gender of a child named "Jane" or "John." Both gender and name are used in Appendix 1c to personalize one of several possible responses to a multiple choice question.

Appendix 2 demonstrates another important form of personalization. The user is asked to choose a pleasurable activity from a short list. That choice permits the next question to refer to that activity rather than a more generic example that might be less attractive.

The commands used to perform some of this processing are shown in Appendix 6. Graphics, sound and animation are added separately to each lesson through Pilot subroutines; TRANS concerns itself primarily with lesson text. Each block of text to appear on a separate screen is started by the #T command (add Text). Text blocks are terminated by #R (press Return to continue); #A (Answer expected); or #M (Match text). #M is similar to #A but permits a word or short phrase to be assigned to a variable based on the answer. #G (Get a subroutine) is one of several ways to include Pilot subroutines. These and other commands are described in Appendix 6.

A portion of a lesson written in TRANS is shown in Appendix 3. The users name has been obtained earlier through a #N command, and was stored in the variable "user." This variable is referred to in all subsequent text as $user$ (a Pilot convention for variable names). At the start of this example, this variable is used to personalize the question text.

The question has four allowed answers: A, B, C, or D. These are automatically inserted in the prompt for this question. The individual responses to each answer are also personalized and the answer are stored for future analysis. Text for questions and responses are centered on the screen. As the example shows, TRANS commands are case insensitive.

Compare this with Appendix 4, the PC Pilot(TM) code output by TRANS. The code shown displays the question and the response to the first choice. It is significantly longer, much more complicated and harder to explain.

Appendix 5 demonstrates how TRANS is used. It first asks a number of questions (Appendix 5a), including the name of the input file containing TRANS code, the name of the file to contain the resulting PC-Pilot(TM) code, whether external PC Pilot(TM) modules are to be included (usually omitted only if they are under development or revision), and questions to determine whether to insert special Pilot code that occurs only at the beginning or end of a lesson. Multipart lessons are easily handled with minor coding at the end and beginning of each part. TRANS requests the number of questions asked in previous parts. It stores all responses to one lesson in one file and sequentially numbers each question, thus needs to know where the numbering left off.

When all questions are answered satisfactorily, TRANS begins (Appendix 5b) its first of up to two passes through the input file. During the first pass, it checks for numerous possible errors, including too many lines for a screen, too many characters for a line, etc. It also sets up tables which will be used to translate TRANS code into Pilot. At the end of the first read, it produces a list of errors. If there are no syntax errors, it will proceed to the next stage.

In the second pass, it rereads the input file and writes the output (Pilot) file. When it completes its translation into Pilot, it outputs how many questions were asked (the number to use when the next piece of the lesson is given to TRANS) and ends. The 687 lines of LESSON1A are thus TRANSlated into 1406 lines of Pilot code.

TRANS Evaluation

TRANS was used to author 10 of the 11 lessons. The only lesson not written or rewritten in TRANS was the second lesson, which was written in Pilot. A total of over 600 hours of programmer and health professional time was spent to produce this 30-minute Pilot lesson.

TRANS significantly shortened lesson production time. The 10 TRANS lessons were produced over a period of 2 years by one half time FTE graduate student programmer and approximately 10-25% FTE health professional time. Thus, approximately 10 weeks and 240-300 hours were invested in each lesson.

However TRANS was NOT used directly by health professionals. Our health professional (SP) could not devote enough time to TRANS to become proficient with it. Instead lesson text would be generated on a typewriter or in long-hand for entry into TRANS by the programmer. Modifications were frequently hand-written on a copy of printed TRANS code.

DISCUSSION

Development Time

As mentioned in the Introduction, the first two lessons of the eleven lessons were already developed before TRANS. The first lesson, written in BASIC, was rewritten in TRANS. However STEP, the second lesson, initially written in Apple Super Pilot(TM) and moved to PC Pilot(TM), was left as it was. The 600 hours used to develop STEP can be contrasted with the 240-300 hours for the lessons developed by TRANS.

Some of the time savings with TRANS is due to increasing familiarity with CAI and the development of standard ways to begin and end lessons. Indeed the amount of time needed for each TRANS lesson decreased during the development period.

Some time savings also is due to restrictions placed on lessons by TRANS. For example, TRANS makes it easy to enter screens of text separated by full-screen graphics; the TRANS lessons thus have fewer graphics intermixed with text on the same screen than the Pilot lesson.

However, TRANS facilitates lesson development in other ways. It permits the programmer to simply enter large amounts of text and produce well-formatted screens with a minimum of effort. Then, while the health professional is examining and revising this text, the programmer can be working on graphics and other special Pilot features to add to the lesson.

Other Benefits of TRANS

There is always "one last typo." These can easily be corrected in the TRANS code without need of a skilled Pilot programmer.

Similarly, whole sections of TRANS code (for lesson evaluation or standard questions) can be moved from one lesson to another. The TRANS ability to work with a lesson in multiple parts permitted the evaluation section to be the last part of most lessons, moved en toto from one lesson to the other.

TRANS code is straight ASCII text with minor control codes (see Appendix 3). This has two major implications for our project. First, the TRANS text file was easily converted into written lessons with the same lesson content. Our project involves evaluating the lessons in both forms, written and computer, and the ease of transfer from one to the other was very helpful.

Finally, one or more of our lessons already have been moved from one computer language to another (BASIC to Pilot) or from one computer system to another (Apple II to IBM PC). Enough time and effort has been invested in these lessons that we may very well want to move them to still other languages or computers in the future. All that would be required is a new TRANS program or procedure, one that takes TRANS code and generates code in the new language and/or for the new computer.

Limitations

Even with TRANS, it still took over 200 hours to produce a 30 minute lesson, or 400 hours per lesson-hour produced. This is significantly more than the 130 hours estimated to produce an hour of CAI for students in the health professions (Pengov, 1978). CAI for the general public on topics in behavioral health education is difficult. Experienced counselors have to adapt their techniques for one-on-one counseling to the new methodology. In addition, there are no standard syllabi, or even standard criteria on what should be taught or learned.

TRANS itself has certain limitations. Though TRANS permits all features of PILOT to be used in a lesson, the features it supports most easily will be most commonly used. This has been noted above as "restrictions" TRANS may place on a lesson. Whether this is a drawback or not depends on whether a lesson suffers from lack of a specific feature. We believe the lessons we produced with TRANS are not inferior to the one produced directly in Pilot.

TRANS however was NOT used directly by the health professional who authored our lessons. These people are very busy and if computer resources are not available exactly when they have free time (perhaps at home or because a patient cancels an appointment on short notice), it is not surprising they will fall back on handwriting or a typewriter to generate lesson text. We still believe that TRANS would be useable by non-computer-oriented personnel given sufficient computer resources and priority for its use.

A final limitation has more to do with advances in technology than TRANS itself. TRANS was developed in 1986, and microcomputers and computer authoring software have advanced since then. For example, one can now purchase an entry-level Macintosh microcomputer system with very high resolution graphics and the Hypercard authoring software for under $1000. Hypercard can introduce graphics, animation, sound and many other special effects into a lesson, and it or similar software would be the language of choice if we were to develop our lessons today.

Future Plans

The lessons that have been developed are being evaluated by parents of children with cystic fibrosis (Petzel et al., 1991a, 1991b). The lessons are being evaluated in both computer and written form. Preliminary results indicate that the computer lessons are as much or more acceptable to the parents than the written lessons.

Since lessons designed for this study must be presented in both written and computer form, they do not use the full power of computer assisted instruction. We would like to enhance one or more of the computer lessons in this series and compare their acceptability to the original lessons. A pilot project to do so in conjunction with translating the lessons into Hypercard(TM) on a Macintosh(TM) computer is underway with the collaboration of M.A. Gillispie of Moorhead State University.

CONCLUSIONS

We have developed TRANS, a PC Pilot preprocessor customized for the development of behavioral health education material. TRANS code is much easier to produce and two to three times shorter than the equivalent PC-Pilot(TM) code. TRANS code is thus a condensed, simplified lesson format useful for proofreading and discussion with health professionals. TRANS was successfully used to author 11 CAI lessons (5.5 hours) on coping skills for parents of children with cystic fibrosis over a two year period. However, TRANS was not suitable for unassisted use by busy health professionals.

TRADEMARKS

Applesoft BASIC™, Apple II™, Apple SuperPILOT™, Hypercard™ and Macintosh™ are trademarks of the Apple Corporation. IBM PC™ is a trademark of the IBM Corporation. PC-Pilot™ is a trademark of the University of Washington. Microsoft BASIC™ is a trademark of the Microsoft Corporation. EZ-PC™ is a trademark of the Zenith Corporation.

REFERENCES

Burling, T.A., Marotta, T., Gonzalez, R., Moltzen, T.O., Eng, A.M., Schmidt, G.A., Welch. R.L., Ziff, D.C., and Reilly, P.M. (1989) Computerized smoking cessation program for the workside: Treatment outcome and feasibility. *Journal of Consulting and Clinical Psychology*, 57(5), 619-622.

Lambert, M.E., Billings, M. (1991). Harnessing computer technology for behavioral therapy training and research. *Progress in Behavioral Modification*, 27, in press.

Pengov, R. E. (1978). CAI at Ohio State College of Medicine. in DeLand, E (ed) *Information Technology in Health Science Education*, New York: Plenum Press, p. 261.

Petzel, S.v., Ellis, L.B.M., Budd, J.R., Warwick, W.J. (1991a). Cystic fibrosis and behavioral health education: Problem solving for parents. *Pediatrics* (submitted).

Petzel, S.v., Ellis, L.B.M., Budd, J.R., Johnson, Y. (1991b) Microcomputers for behavioral health education: Developing and evaluating patient education for the chronically ill. in Miller, M (ed) *Computer Applications in Mental Health – 1991*. New York: The Haworth Press, Inc., in press.

Schneider, S.T. (1986). Trial of an on-line behavioral smoking cessation program. *Computers in Human Behavior* 2(4), 277-286.

Tombari, M.L., Fitzpatrick, S.T., and Childress, W. (1985). Using computers as contingency managers in self-monitoring interventions: A case study. *Computers in Human Services* 1(1), 75-82.

APPENDIX 1 – LESSON PERSONALIZATION EXAMPLE

a. Is your child a girl or a boy?

   Type g or b > *g*

b. What is her name?

> *Alice*

   .

   .

   .

c. – – Resenting Demands on You – –

A. Tell Alice you don't like the treatment and would rather do something else, but don't make her feel guilty.

APPENDIX 2—LESSON PERSONALIZATION, CON'TD

a. What is one activity you like to do?

A. Reading

B. Watching TV

C. Talking to a friend

Type A, B, or C > *C*

b. When you talk to your friend. . . .

APPENDIX 3—EXAMPLE TRANS LESSON CODE

#T

Thank you, $user$.

In helping you cope with CF, how important do you think it is to know MANY different coping skills?

A. Not really important

B. A little important

C. Moderately important

D. Very important

#A

#ca

$user$, you will be learning how MANY different coping skills can be useful.

#r

#cb

$user$, you will be learning how MANY different coping skills can be useful.

#R

#cc

$user$, you already know it is important to use MANY coping skills. Keep up the good work.

#r

#cd

$user$, you already know it is important to use MANY coping skills. Keep up the good work.

#R

APPENDIX 4—PILOT CODE PRODUCED BY TRANS

*FR6

P:

X:XCLS$

TS:V24, 80, 5, 25

T:Thank you, $user$.

T:

T:

T:In helping you cope with CF, how

T:important do you think it is to

T:know MANY different coping skills?T:

T:

T: A. Not really important

T: B. A little important

T: C. Moderately important

T: D. Very important

T:

T:

TS:V20,80,23,25

TH: >

AS:

```
C:XQUEST = 2

M:a
JN:@M
X:XCLS$
C:XQ$ = ,"!!XQUEST!!","!!%B
C:XP$ = XP$!!XQ$
TS:V22, 80, 10, 25
T:$user$, you will be learning how MANY
T:different coping skills can be useful.
T:
U:HELLO
E:
J:@P
```

APPENDIX 5 — EXAMPLE TRANS RUN

a.

> *basica trans* [Users responses are *underlined.*]

Enter the name of the file you wish to translate: <u>LESSON1A</u>

Enter the name you wish to give the new program [.PIL]:

<u>intro.pil</u>

Do you want to merge the #G subroutines at this time?

  (Y or N) <u>Y</u>

Is this the first or only part of this lesson? (Y or N) <u>Y</u>

[If answer is no] How many questions (#A) do you have in the previous part of this lesson?

Is this the last part of this lesson? (Y or N) <u>N</u>

b.

Reading LESSON1A

Done with 1st read

Number of errors = 0 [if errors, error messages appear here]

Total number of lines in LESSON1A = 687

Writing intro.pil

Finished Merging #G Subroutines

FINISHED WRITING intro.pil

LAST QUESTION # = 11

Press any key to clear screen and return to DOS

APPENDIX 6 – SOME TRANS COMMANDS

#T begins a block of text to appear on one screen.

#R ends a block of text and inserts "Press RETURN to continue."

#A ends a block of text containing a multiple choice or true/false question, including the prompt: "Type x, y, or z," and indicates that allowable answers follow.

#CA one anticipated answer is "A" (upper or lower case) and the text response to that answer follows.

#S ends text that asks a gender determination question and prompts for the answer (a gender designator). M, B, or any word beginning with m or b will change the gender variables to indicate male; F, G, or any word beginning with f or g will change them to indicate female.

#Nnnn ends text that asks a name question, prompts for the answer, and assigns the name string to the variable nnn.

#Mnnn ends a block of text containing a question, prompts for answer just as a #A, and indicates answers follow. Answers will assign a string to the variable nnn.

#CB"watch TV" the string 'watch TV' will be associated with the variable given in the preceding #M

#Gname allows incorporation of external Pilot subroutine "name"

Microcomputers for Behavioral Health Education: Developing and Evaluating Patient Education for the Chronically Ill

Sue V. Petzel
Lynda B. M. Ellis
Jeffrey R. Budd
Y. Johnson

KEYWORDS. Cystic fibrosis, health education, chronic illness, computer-assisted instruction

SUMMARY. Eleven lessons in written and computer formats have been developed to promote self-efficacy and to teach three coping skills: problem solving, social networking, and communication. The lessons are being evaluated by sixty four parents of children with cystic fibrosis. The overall goal of this study is to compare the effectiveness of written lessons, computer lessons and generic mental health materials.

This paper describes the lesson series and the evaluation of the

---

Sue V. Petzel, PhD, is a staff psychologist at the Health Psychology Clinic, University of Minnesota, Box 731 UMHC, Minneapolis, MN 55455.

The authors thank the staff, patients and patient families of the University of Minnesota Regional Cyctic Fibrosis Clinic for their continuing help in this study. They thank Ya-Jung Tsai, MS for initial data analyses and Susan Kujawa, RN for study coordination and patient liaison activities. The authors also thank Paul Welle, MD and Lily Chen for assistance with lesson development and Janelle Hammond, Laurie Maneutfel, and Royal Becker for assistance with patient recruitment, testing and delivery of lessons. This study was supported in part by NIH DER HL37504-01. Write to the author for information on software availability.

fourth and fifth lessons. Preliminary results indicate the computer lessons are as or more acceptable than written lessons or generic health education brochures. Lessons, unlike brochures, are rated increasingly more favorably as more are completed. Parents completing lessons four (p < 0.001) and five (p = 0.015) in computer form rate themselves as learning significantly more than those completing the corresponding written lessons and brochures.

Computer-assisted instruction emphasizing the active acquisition of coping skills and promoting self-efficacy is well received by parents of children with cystic fibrosis and can be rated more highly than written lessons or generic mental health brochures.

BACKGROUND

Cystic fibrosis (CF) is the most common lethal genetic disease of Caucasian children. Its prevalence is approximately 1 in 2000 live births in the United States (Wood et al., 1976). Despite advances in medical therapies and dramatically improved survival, CF is characterized by progressive deterioration in lung and gastrointestinal functions. While the majority of patients with CF survive into their mid-30's, extensive therapeutic efforts slow but do not eliminate the disease (Zach, 1990).

Cystic fibrosis has changed from a fatal pediatric illness to a chronic disability impacting patients and their families for decades. It has been described as a prototype condition for the study of stress in families with chronically ill children (Walker et al., 1987). Efforts to facilitate psychosocial adaption take on increased relevance as mortality declines. Increasingly, for children and adults with CF, research and clinical practice have emphasized ways to strengthen psychosocial adaption (Mattsson, 1977) and to identify and reduce adaptive problems (Petzel et al., 1984). However, while systematic efforts to promote psychosocial adaptation for this expanding population have been recommended, program development and outcome research are limited.

Conceptual Models

Research with a variety of pediatric health problems other than CF suggests psychosocial interventions based on patient education, social learning and family system models can be developed to meet a broad range of psychosocial and health care needs.

Research has demonstrated the value of patient education as a significant part of routine pediatric health care and an integral part of coping with chronic childhood health conditions, such as asthma (Evans et al., 1990; Nader, 1985; Thoresen and Kirmil-Gray, 1985). Advantages of adding an educational component to the medical model include the focus on health rather than disease; the de-emphasis on a simplistic view of illness; the assumption that the patient and clinician both have power; and the support of an active role for the patient and the patient's family (Bartlett, EE, 1985). In the management of CF, a health education approach can be used to promote new health behaviors as well as increase knowledge and change attitudes for children and family members.

An educational model places an emphasis on learning and the application of learning principles. Accepted learning principles include use of reinforcement, especially immediate positive rewards; and use of homework, contracts and tutorials. Principles of effective health education recommend therapists: specify patient behaviors desired and the obstacles to these; individualize and personalize education; include instructional (information/knowledge) and behavioral (i.e., what to do) strategies; attend to long-term performance of desired behaviors; and facilitate developing the patient's social support (Bartlett, 1985).

In addition to traditional learning and health educational principles for patients and their families, Bandura's social learning theory has demonstrated particular usefulness in designing health behavior change programs. A critical cognitive component in social learning theory is the concept of self-efficacy, the level of conviction that one is capable of doing certain things which influence choices, effort levels and persistence (Bandura, 1982). Perceptions of self-efficacy are hypothesized to affect how much effort people will extend and how long they will persist in the face of obstacles or adverse experiences. Self-efficacy judgements also mediate the quality of one's emotional reaction. Self-efficacy has been demonstrated to be strongly associated with health behavior change (O'Leary, 1985; Strecher, DeVellis, Beaker, & Rosenstock, 1986) and to be an important motivational factor in medical adherence (Evans et al., 1990).

Families with children who have CF have a central role in providing for their child's daily health care and treatment (Walker et al., 1987; Patterson, 1985). The subsequent demands and stresses on the family and the child can result in behavioral problems for young patients and increased family dysfunction (Cowan et al., 1986). Therefore, it is important to attend to both the child and the family's needs in designing behavioral health interventions for this chronic care population.

Family involvement in health behavior change programs represents several significant possibilities. A family-based intervention has the potential for training and motivating multiple family members; attempts to minimize possible barriers posed by family members; and trains a variety of social supports with the family to enhance the behavioral change process. Theoretically such training could lead to greater and broader social behavior change (Baranowski and Nader, 1985).

Combining the educational, social learning and family behavior change models to design an intervention program for the CF population results in the following recommendations: (a) use accepted learning principles, (b) promote information acquisition and skill development and maintenance, (c) include active family involvement, (d) promote self-efficacy, (e) individualize and personalize instruction, and (f) build social support.

All three models recognize the value of skill development. While this is an essential ingredient in developing intervention programs, these models do not specify which skills are to be taught or what modality of instruction is to be used.

Computer-Assisted Instruction to Teach Coping Skills

There is no agreement on a minimum set of requisite skills to cope with chronic disease. However, research has identified eleven generic coping skills commonly used by parents of children with CF to cope with the variety of problems and stresses they experience. Communication, problem solving, and social networking are three skills used particularly frequently by these parents (Petzel et al., 1984). Not surprisingly, these skills have been demonstrated repeatedly to be of value in coping with other serious health problems for both chronically ill children and adults (Ewart, 1990; Moos, 1977).

However, limited research has occurred on the design and evaluation of materials to teach these coping skills to the chronically-ill, including those with CF. Traditionally, small group or one-on-one interaction has been used to teach complex problem solving, social skills and communication techniques to individuals. Often such intensive, long-term interventions are ineffective due to limited participation: the individuals being counseled miss their appointments or only passively attend. Such interventions also are professionally labor-intensive; frequently financially costly; and often are delivered on a selective and reactive, rather than systematic and preventative, basis.

A variety of computerized treatment protocols have been developed either to provide complex skill training or as adjunctive enhancements to non-computer-based treatment efforts (Lambert and Billings, 1991). Computer-assisted instruction (CAI) has the potential to provide skill training without the limitations of small group or one-on-one presentations. The computer lessons can be presented at times more convenient to the client, which may motivate client participation. The computer also can be an active, individualized form of instruction, challenging passive participation.

Research and development of computer applications in health care have focused on the management of medical data, e.g., medical record systems; medical decision making; and medical education (Shortliffe et al., 1990). However, health educators, recognizing the potential of microcomputers, are beginning to develop guidelines for developing health education software (for example, Horne and Gold, 1983). Encouraging results include: CAI has been found to be a cost-effective method of health education; has been positively accepted by patients with cystic fibrosis; and adult users self-report willingness to change health behavior due to a CAI lesson, especially in populations with increased risk of poor health behaviors (Ellis et al., 1982, 1983). Advantages of CAI include its ability to provide individualized instruction, continuous feedback to the learner about performance, documentation of an individual's performance, and storage of an individual's responses for later retrieval.

The potential of CAI for health education and the need of families with chronically-ill children to develop coping skills led to our study of CAI to teach coping skills to parents of children with CF. Consistent with a health education and social learning perspective, the lessons are intended to teach concepts, skills and attitudes, including self-efficacy. This report is the latest in a series on this project; an earlier report includes citations on its history (Petzel et al., 1991).

MATERIALS AND METHODS

Study Population

As previously discussed in more detail (Petzel et al., 1991), parents of 52 CF children (27 boys, 25 girls) from 6 months to eleven years of age were asked to volunteer for this study. Parents were selected from 101 families with children in this age range who are routinely followed at the University of Minnesota Regional Cystic Fibrosis Clinic for regular care. Each parent signs a consent form and is assigned randomly to one of three groups to receive either computer lessons, written lessons, or generic mental health brochures.

Prior to receiving lessons or brochures, parents complete baseline standardized tests. Testing will be repeated following completion of all 11 interventions. The 51 mothers and 16 fathers who completed evaluations had a mean age of 35.4 years.

While in this study, all participating parents rate their own stress levels using a ten-item checklist and monitor their child's health status. These records are sent to the clinic monthly. The child's health status also is monitored by health care professionals as part of their regular quarterly clinic visit.

Lessons

Eleven lessons teaching coping skills to parents of children with chronic illness or disability were developed as previously reported (Petzel et al., 1991; Ellis et al., 1991). These lessons emphasize identifying problems and learning and practicing problem solving, social networking and communication skills. Within these lessons, self-efficacy is promoted by guiding users through problem situations and learning tasks. Users encounter corrective feedback and vicarious modeling in which they observe desired behavior; for example, users follow a hypothetical parent through successful task/problem completion. Lessons also include rehearsing cognitions regarding self-efficacy; e.g., positive self-statements such as "I am confident setting goals helps me succeed in solving problems."

Each lesson is designed to take approximately 30 minutes and is aimed at a 6-8th grade reading level. The Flesch-Kincaid test as implemented in Grammatik Mac 1.0 (Anon., 1990) was used to rate reading level. The first four lessons had a level of 6-8th grade and the fifth lesson had a level of 5th grade.

The lessons were developed using PC Pilot and a locally written software package called TRANS, as described previously (Ellis et al., 1991). The computer lessons were developed and used on an IBM-compatible Zenith EZ-PC with a 20 Mbyte hard disk drive and monochrome, CGA monitor.

After each computer lesson was developed, it was reformatted for use as a written lesson. Time and detailed attention were given to the development and production of both the written and computer materials. This included repeated review of both sets of materials by staff and by patients not directly involved in the study. Thus, written and computer lessons were designed to have equivalent content, conceptualization, and production quality.

Examples of lesson content are shown in Figures 1 and 2. Figure 1 presents an introductory display from Lesson 5, demonstrating the

Figure 1 - An introductory display from Lesson 5

The goals of this lesson are to teach you:

    what is a support network,

    .
    what is YOUR support network, and

    .
    how strong is YOUR support network.

You will look as three key WAYS to find out how strong your support is, and use a worksheet to look at the strength of your support.

Press <Return> to continue.

Figure 2 - Example of Content Flow in Lesson 5

(Words in parentheses are not shown on
the screen. $user$ = user's name)

Now, $user$, think of some people who
either advise or help you NOW.

Who is your closest FRIEND?

Type in the person's first name or nickname
below. Type N if there is no one. If you
mistype, press the Back Space key and make
corrections. When finished, press <RETURN>.

(Similar questions elucidate names of a helpful NEIGHBOR, RELATIVE, person who
helps with PERSONAL PROBLEMS, CO-WORKER or FELLOW STUDENT, and an EXPERT. The
answers to these six questions may include multiple instances of the same
person, the N indicating "no one", or two or more people with the same first
name.)

(Summary)
(Answer Names are repeated)

Looking at these names, how many
different people did you list?

A. no one
B. one or two
C. three or more

Choose A, B, or C.
(Reinforcement)

(Answer A or B): You are being helped by very few
                  people. This lesson may suggest
                  ways to increase this number.

                  (You need more LINKS).

(Answer C): You are helped by several different people.
                  (You have several LINKS in your network.)

                  That's GOOD!

                  Press <Return> to continue.

(Instructional Feedback)

A network is made up of many links. Each
link supports each of the other links. . . .

description of the goals of the lesson and what is expected as part of completing the lesson. Figure 2 presents an example of content flow from Lesson 5. The topics of the first five lessons are shown in Table 1.

The content of the first three lessons have been previously described (Petzel et al., 1991). Lesson 4 includes setting goals for problems and working towards these goals. Lesson 5 introduces the concept of support networks, including their value in times of physical illness, and how to identify the strength of each individual's own social network.

All lessons include worksheets which are homework assignments that the parent completes and mails back to the clinic. Worksheets promote practicing coping skills in the parent's home environment and encourage generalization of skills from the clinic to "real life." The lessons and worksheets emphasize positive reinforcement of concepts; instructional feedback; skill rehearsal; and are designed to strengthen parents' self-efficacy; that is, their knowledge that they are competent to handle a range of problems and stresses through effective use of a variety of skills. The lessons also support an educational model of health care (Bartlett, 1985). Frequency of worksheet return will be used, at the end of the study, as one measure of compliance.

The 11 generic mental health brochures include pamphlets or articles on parenting, stress management, and other topics. Mental health materials selected for use were intended to be well-conceptualized and produced; informative; readily available; and present concepts of recognized and reputable merit. These materials are not specific to chronic illness. For example, the fourth examines how to

Table 1 - The First Five Lessons

1.	Coping Skills for Families: Problem Solving in Chronic Illness
2.	A S.T.E.P. to Problem Solving
3.	S.T.E.P. Ahead - Managing Stress
4.	STEPping Toward Your Goals
5.	PEOPLE CAN BE GOOD MEDICINE: Building Social Connections

handle stress (Lerner and Elins, 1985); and the fifth, four fact sheets from the Association for Advancement of Behavioral Therapy, discusses the common complaints depression, insomnia, alcohol abuse and headache (Anon. 1988a,b; 1989a,b). No worksheets accompany the generic mental health brochures.

Evaluation

Eleven lessons, one or two at a time, are completed by parents during routine quarterly clinic visits. At a projected rate of two lessons per visit, a parent would complete all eleven in six visits, or approximately 18 months. Parents receive lessons (or brochures) in the clinic waiting room on the day their child is seen for a routine, pre-scheduled appointment. After completing a lesson or brochure, parents evaluate it by answering three questions (Figure 3).

Statistics

A t test is used to compare the answers to evaluation questions regarding individual lessons between two groups: computer lessons and written lessons or brochure.

Figure 3 - Evaluation Questions to be Completed Following Lesson Use

---

How helpful was this lesson to you?

    1.   Not helpful, a waste of time
    2.   Slightly helpful
    3.   Moderately helpful
    4.   Very helpful, I'd recommend it

Will you change any living habits because of this lesson?

    1.   Definitely not
    2.   Probably not
    3.   Perhaps
    4.   Probably yes
    5.   Definitely yes

How much did you learn?

    1.   Almost nothing
    2.   A little
    3.   Some
    4.   Moderate amount
    5.   Considerable

RESULTS

Evaluation

Evaluation data for lessons 1-3 and preliminary data for lesson 4 have been reported previously (Petzel et al., 1991). Here we report on more detailed analysis of lesson 4 and lesson 5.

The evaluation data for lessons and brochures 1 throu h 5 are shown in Table 2. The three evaluation questions shown in Figure 3 are summarized as Help?, Change?, and Learn? and numbers under those headings are the means of the coded answers. Computer and written lesson evaluations are compared in Figure 4.

For all three ratings by parents, later computer lessons were rated more highly than earlier lessons for the first four lessons, and appear to have stabilized at a high level for lesson five. This effect

Table 2 - Self-Reported Lesson Evaluation[a]

Intervention	Type[b]	N	Help?	Change?	Learn?	p Value[c]
Lesson 1	C	29	2.9	3.2	3.2	0.007
	W	26	2.6	2.8	2.4	
	B	11	3.1	3.5	2.9	
Lesson 2	C	24	3.0	3.4	3.8	<0.001
	W	24	2.7	2.9	2.7	
	B	20	2.6	3.3	2.6	
Lesson 3	C	18	3.2	3.7	3.6	0.004
	W	14	2.7	3.1	2.7	
	B	7	2.6	2.8	2.4	
Lesson 4	C	14	3.5	3.9	4.1	<0.001
	W	12	3.0	3.8	2,9	
	B	11	3.1	3.7	2.6	
Lesson 5	C	8	3.5	3.5	4.0	0.015
	W	11	3.2	3.2	3.1	
	B	7	2.6	3.1	2.4	

a. Data for lessons 1-3 are as previously reported (Petzel et al., 1991).
b. C = Computer Lesson, W = Written Lesson, B = Brochure
c. Significance level of difference in Amount Learned rating between computer and written lessons for lessons 1-3; between computer lessons and written lessons or brochures for lessons 4-5.

was smaller for written lessons, and was nonexistent for generic mental health brochures (Table 2).

DISCUSSION

Lesson Development

Eleven lessons were developed and are now being evaluated. Lesson development was slower than expected. Three main reasons for this slow development were difficulty in using a general purpose authoring language which required development of our own PC Pilot preprocessor (Ellis et al., 1991), lack of a defined syllabus (discussed in Ellis et al., 1991), and limitations of using a 6-8th grade reading level for lessons.

Families are drawn from a wide variety of socioeconomic backgrounds and education levels. Parents thus have varying reading levels, and pretest screening included a reading level test. All parents screened achieved at least a 6th grade reading level, the lowest target level of our lessons. No parent was excluded from the study because of low literacy.

Minnesota and the upper midwest region have relatively high literacy levels and rates of graduation from high school. In other populations, lessons at even lower literacy levels might be required. This might necessitate quite different educational approaches, perhaps using audio tapes or more visual means of communication, since lessons at levels below 6th grade are usually too simplistic for more advanced readers.

Developing materials to be understood at even the 6-8th grade reading level was confining. Many of the concepts to be taught are abstract or include medical or health terminology, requiring words not at an elementary reading level. The format of the computer screen also is restricting, requiring shorter words and sentences than the equivalent material in written form.

Study Population

The lessons which were specifically developed for this study focus on issues that are potentially sensitive and highly personal, such as intimate relationships, death and dying, and family conflict.

Thus it is useful to document that parents are compliant with the tasks required of them as part of this study: they are willing to participate and cooperate with study testing and methodology. This is important given the challenges of lesson development and evaluation.

Study Environment

Lessons and brochures in this study were originally planned to be offered to parents in a separate, parent education center adjacent to the clinic waiting area. Unfortunately, use of such a center was not available. Thus lessons were completed by parents in the clinic waiting room or a hall alcove.

Parents often report experiencing high stress in this clinical environment. This included difficulty concentrating on lessons, even when the lessons were described as interesting and valuable. A separate room might mitigate, but probably not eliminate, this problem. Often the stress is associated with the clinic appointment itself. Each appointment includes the possibility of many stressful events, such as documentation of a child's deteriorating health, physician reminders of the need for therapy, fear that the visit will uncover unknown problems, and issues associated with adherence.

The potentially distracting effects of the clinic environment were underestimated in planning the implementation of the study. Home use of lessons or use in separate sessions not related to medical visits may facilitate more effective learning.

Lesson Evaluation

In an analysis of variance taking into account the format of the material (computer or non-computer) and the type of the material (lesson or brochure), the computer lessons were rated higher than written lessons or brochures for all three evaluation questions for the first three lessons. This difference was statistically significant for self-reported amount learned. The type of material did not play a significant role in any of the ratings (Petzel et al., 1991). Similarly, in the present analysis of lessons 4 and 5, parents reported learning more from the computer lesson format than from the written format.

Results in the present paper are based upon self-reported evaluations. Such evaluations are not expected to replace measures of behavior change, such as increase in coping skills, decrease in stress levels, or increased compliance. Measures of these outcome indices will be determined after parents have completed all 11 lessons and are retested. The self-reported evaluations of non-specific (generic) brochures will be used as a minimum standard for our specific lessons.

Results for the first two lessons indicate the computer lessons are as acceptable or more acceptable to the parents, as shown by helpfulness, intent to change, and amount learned ratings, as written lessons or generic mental health brochures (Petzel et al., 1991). Also, for each individual lesson, parents self-report learning significantly more from the material in computer format than from the corresponding lesson in written format. There are no significant differences between the ratings of written lessons and generic health education brochures.

Active participation in a lesson via computer may facilitate learning compared to more passive written lessons, even though the latter were developed in workbook format, with many questions to be answered. This is supported by the increase in self-reported "amount learned" in computer lessons as compared with written lessons.

Psychological interventions provide ways to cope with what traditionally have been considered medical problems. Increasingly health psychology research has recognized the value of multidimensional programs which incorporate diverse therapeutic components in the treatment of chronic disease (Genest and Genest, 1987).

The present study includes efforts designed to influence the ways in which parents think, and to promote the active acquisition of multiple coping skills and generalization and maintenance of these skills within daily life. Parent participation and evaluation in this study suggests this special population of parents is ready for innovative and multidimensional efforts targeted at health promotion and health behavior change, and that CAI has a promising role in this process. Study completion will help to identify which parents are more and less likely to be helped by behavioral health education so as to maximize treatment benefits.

CONCLUSIONS

Computer-assisted instruction emphasizing the acquisition of multiple coping skills and promoting self-efficacy is well received by parents of children with cystic fibrosis. Lessons specifically designed for this population and teaching a given coping skill such as problem solving can be rated more highly than generic mental health brochures and promote an increasingly favorable response as an increasing number of lessons are completed. Lessons presented in computer form are rated significantly higher in "amount learned" than corresponding lessons in written form.

However, developing lessons to promote behavior change at a minimal literacy level is challenging and time-consuming. Lesson delivery within a demanding clinic routine and in competition with serious health care needs may compromise effective implementation and may delay efficient knowledge acquisition. These factors may in part explain the present dearth of CAI for patient education, even given its apparent value.

REFERENCES

Anonymous (1988a) Depression. New York: Association for Advancement of Behavioral Therapy.

Anonymous (1988b) Headache. New York:Association for Advancement of Behavioral Therapy.

Anonymous (1989a) Insomnia. New York:Association for Advancement of Behavioral Therapy.

Anonymous (1989b) Alcohol Abuse. New York: Association for Advancement of Behavioral Therapy.

Anonymous (1990), Grammatik Mac User's Guide, version 1.0, San Francisco Reference Software International.

Bandura, A. (1982) Self-efficacy mechanisms in human agency. American Psychologist 37:122-147.

Baranowski, T and Nader, P.R. (1985) A Life-Span Perspective in Turk, D. and Kerns, R (eds) Family Involvement in Health Behavior Change Programs. New York: John Wiley and Sons.

Bartlett EE (1985) Patient education introduction: Eight principles from patient education research. Preventive Medicine 14:667-669.

Cowan L, Mok J, Corey M, MacMillan H, Simmons R, Levison H (1986) Psychological adjustment of the family with a member who has cystic fibrosis. Pediatrics 77:745-753.

Ellis LBM, Raines JR, Hakanson N (1982) Health education using microcomputers: One year in the clinic. Preventive Medicine 11:212-223.

Ellis LBM, Petzel Sv, Asp EH (1983) Computer-assisted instruction for the chronically-ill child. Proceedings of the 7th Annual Symposium on Computer Applications in Medical Care. New York, Institute of Electrical and Electronic Engineers, pp. 366-369.

Ellis LBM., Welle P, and Petzel Sv. (1991) A pilot preprocessor for patient education. in M. Miller (ed) Proceedings of the Conference on Computer Applications in Mental Health – 1991 Update, Indianapolis, in press.

Evans, D., Clarck, N.M., Feldman, X., Wasilewski, Y., Levin, B., and Mellins, R.B. (1990) In Schumaker, S.A., Schron, E.B. and Ockeve, J.K. (eds) The Handbook of Health Behavior Change. New York: Springer.

Ewart CK (1990) A social problem-solving approach to behavior change in coronary heart disease. In Schumaker SA, Schron EB, Ockeve JK (eds): The Handbook of Health Behavior Change. New York, Springer Publishing Co.

Genest M, Genest S (1987) Psychological intervention in physical disorders. in Psychology and Health. Champaign, Illinois: Research Press.

Horne DA, Gold RS: Guidelines for developing health education software. Health Education 1983;10:85.

Lambert ME and Billings M (1991) Harnessing computer technology for behavioral therapy: Training and research. Progress in Behavioral Modification 27. in press.

Lerner H, Elins R (1985) Stress Breakers. Minneapolis: CompCare Publications.

Mattsson A (1977) Long-term physical illness in childhood: A challenge to psychosocial adaptation. In Moos RH (ed): Coping with Physical Illness. New York, Plenum.

Moos, R.H. (ed) (1977) Coping with Physical Illness. New York: Plenum Press.

Nader PR (1985) Improving the practice of pediatric patient education: A synthesis and selective review. Preventive Medicine 14:688-701.

O'Leary (1985) Self-efficacy and health. Behavioral Research and Therapy 23: 437-451.

Patterson JM (1985) Critical factors affecting family compliance with home treatment for children with cystic fibrosis. Family Relations 34:79-89.

Petzel Sv, Bugge I, Warwick WJ, Budd JR (1984) Long term adaptation of children and adolescents with cystic fibrosis: Identification of common problems and risk factors. In Blum RW (ed): Chronic Illness and Disabilities in Childhood and Adolescence. New York, Grune & Stratton, 1984, pp. 413-427.

Petzel Sv, Ellis LBM, Budd JR., Warwick, WJ (1991).Cystic Fibrosis and Behavioral Health Education:Problem Solving for Parents Pediatrics, submitted.

Shortliffe, E. H., Perreault, L. E., Wiederhold, G., & Fagan, L. M. (1990). Medical Informatics: Computer applications in health care. N.Y.: Addison-Wesley Publishing Company.

Streacher, V.J, DeVillis, B.M., Becher, M.A., and Rosestock, I.M. (1986). The role of self-efficacy in achieving health behavior change. Health Education Quarterly 13 73-91.

Thoresen CE, Kirmil-Gray K (1985) Self-management psychology and the treatment of childhood asthma. Journal Allergy Clin Immunology 1985;72:596-606.

Walker LS, Ford MB, Donald WD (1987) Cystic fibrosis and family stress: Effects of age and severity of illness. Pediatrics 9:239-246.

Wood RE, Boat TF, Doershuk CF (1976) Cystic fibrosis. Am Rev Respir Dis 113:833-878.

Zach MS (1990) Lung disease in cystic fibrosis – An updated concept. Ped Pulmonol 8:188-202.

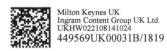